The Complete DASH Diet Cookbook for Seniors

2000 Days of Delicious, Heart-Healthy, Easy-to-Prepare Low-Sodium Recipes to Lower Blood Pressure and Support Weight Loss. Includes a 30-Day Meal Plan.

Amanda K. Sanders

Table of Contents

Introduction

Welcome to *"The Complete DASH Diet Cookbook for Seniors,"* a comprehensive guide to adopting a delicious, anti-hypertensive diet tailored to the needs of older adults. As we age, our nutritional requirements evolve, and it's crucial to adhere to a diet that fosters our overall health, helps manage chronic conditions, and encourages a long and fulfilling life. The DASH diet, which stands for Dietary Approaches to Stop Hypertension, is a scientifically proven approach to eating that can help you achieve these objectives.

Why the DASH Diet?

The DASH diet was initially created to address high blood pressure, but its benefits go well beyond that. By emphasizing whole, nutrient-dense foods and reducing sodium intake, the DASH diet can improve heart health, support bone density, improve cognitive function, and boost overall vitality. This diet is beneficial for seniors as it effectively tackles numerous health issues commonly linked to aging, including hypertension, heart disease, osteoporosis, and diabetes.

What to Expect from This Cookbook

This cookbook is designed to ensure that you can effortlessly integrate the DASH diet into your everyday routine. Inside, you will find:

- A comprehensive overview of the DASH Diet: Learn about the principles and benefits of the DASH diet and how it can support your overall well-being and vitality as you age.
- Meal Planning and Preparation Tips: Find practical advice on how to effectively plan your meals, shop for groceries, and create mouthwatering DASH-friendly dishes.
- A Wide Range of Recipes: This cookbook provides a diverse selection of nutritious and easy recipes, covering everything from filling breakfasts to satisfying dinners, snacks, and desserts.
- Tips for Healthy Aging: Discover ways to maintain an active lifestyle, stay hydrated, and be mindful of your eating habits, all of which can contribute to a healthier and more fulfilling life.

Getting the DASH Diet to Work for You

Rather than impose strict rules or cause deprivation, the DASH diet focuses on helping you make intelligent, sustainable food choices with some flexibility to fit your lifestyle and preferences. If you're new to the DASH diet or want to expand your knowledge further, this cookbook offers the resources and motivation necessary for success.

Here are some helpful tips to get you started:

- Start Slow: Gradually introduce more DASH-friendly foods into your meals. Start by including an extra serving of vegetables or transitioning to whole grains.
- Experiment with Flavors: Incorporate herbs and spices into your cooking to boost the flavor of your meals without relying on excessive sodium.
- Stay Flexible: The DASH diet is highly versatile and can be adjusted to accommodate a wide range of dietary needs and preferences. Feel free to adjust recipes to better match your preferences and dietary needs.

Embrace a Healthier Future

Embracing the DASH diet will improve your heart health and overall wellness. This cookbook is your trusted companion, offering numerous mouthwatering recipes and invaluable insights to support your success.

Thank you for selecting "The Ultimate DASH Diet Cookbook for Seniors." We hope you find joy and inspiration in these pages and that this cookbook proves to be a valuable resource in your journey toward a healthier and happier self.

Chapter 1: Discovering the DASH Diet: A Path to Better Health for Seniors

What is the DASH Diet?

The "DASH" acronym stands for Dietary Approaches to Stop Hypertension. It's a flexible, balanced eating plan designed to boost heart health and lower blood pressure. It's all about enjoying whole foods packed with essential nutrients while cutting back on sodium and unhealthy fats. The DASH diet can be a game-changer for seniors, offering a practical, sustainable way to eat that enhances overall health and vitality.

The DASH diet emphasizes nutrient-rich foods like fruits, vegetables, whole grains, lean proteins, and low-fat dairy products. These foods contain vitamins, minerals, and antioxidants that keep your body running smoothly and help protect against chronic diseases. By reducing sodium and making heart-healthy choices, the DASH diet is particularly effective at managing hypertension, a common issue among older adults.

Why the DASH Diet is Great for Seniors

The DASH diet brings many benefits, especially for seniors facing various age-related health challenges. Here are some key advantages:

1. **Managing Blood Pressure**: One of the biggest perks of the DASH diet is its ability to lower blood pressure. It emphasizes potassium-rich foods like fruits and vegetables while reducing sodium intake, helping to balance electrolyte levels and combat hypertension.

2. **Improving Heart Health**: The DASH diet supports heart health by promoting whole grains, lean proteins, and healthy fats from sources like nuts and olive oil. These foods help lower cholesterol levels and reduce the risk of heart disease, which is crucial for seniors.

3. **Supporting Bone Health**: As we age, keeping our bones strong is vital. The DASH diet includes foods high in calcium and vitamin D, such as low-fat dairy products and leafy greens, which support bone density and reduce the risk of osteoporosis.

4. **Enhancing Overall Well-being**: The DASH diet focuses on whole, unprocessed foods, ensuring a rich intake of essential nutrients. This balanced approach can lead to improved energy levels, better digestion, and a stronger immune system—all important for healthy aging.

Key Nutrients in the DASH Diet

For seniors, getting enough key nutrients is essential for maintaining health and vitality. The DASH diet excels in providing these crucial nutrients:

1. **Calcium**: Critical for bone health, calcium helps prevent osteoporosis and keeps bones strong. Calcium is present in low-fat dairy products, leafy green vegetables, and fortified plant-based milks.

2. **Potassium:** This vital mineral helps regulate blood pressure by counteracting the effects of sodium. Potassium-rich foods include bananas, sweet potatoes, beans, and leafy greens—all staples of the DASH diet.

3. **Magnesium**: Important for muscle and nerve function, magnesium also supports heart health and bone strength. Nuts, seeds, whole grains, and green leafy vegetables are excellent sources of magnesium.

4. **Fiber**: A high-fiber diet aids digestion, helps control blood sugar levels, and supports heart health. The DASH diet includes a variety of fiber-rich foods like fruits, vegetables, whole grains, and legumes, contributing to overall digestive health and well-being.

By focusing on these key nutrients, the DASH diet not only addresses specific health concerns for seniors but also promotes a comprehensive approach to healthy aging. Embracing the DASH diet can significantly improve quality of life, making it an ideal choice for seniors looking to boost their health with balanced and nutritious eating.

Chapter 2: 30-Day Meal Plan

Days 1-10

Day	Breakfast	Lunch	Dinner	Snacks
1	Mediterranean Egg White Omelette (Page 9)	Greek Salad with Quinoa (Page 46)	Grilled Lemon Herb Chicken (Page 65)	Hummus and Veggie Stuffed Cucumber (Page 83)
2	Quinoa and Vegetable Breakfast Bowl (Page 10)	Avocado and Chickpea Salad (Page 47)	Baked Salmon with Dill Sauce (Page 66)	Greek Yogurt and Berry Popsicles (Page 84)
3	Berry Chia Seed Pudding (Page 11)	Spinach and Strawberry Salad (Page 48)	Turkey and Quinoa Stuffed Peppers (Page 67)	Roasted Chickpeas with Herbs (Page 85)
4	Spinach and Feta Breakfast Wrap (Page 12)	Cucumber and Tomato Salad with Feta (Page 49)	Eggplant and Lentil Moussaka (Page 68)	Edamame and Sea Salt Snack (Page 86)
5	Smoked Salmon Avocado Toast (Page 13)	Tuna and White Bean Salad (Page 50)	Shrimp and Vegetable Stir-Fry (Page 69)	Whole Grain Pita with Tzatziki (Page 87)
6	Greek Yogurt Parfait with Mixed Berries (Page 14)	Quinoa and Black Bean Salad (Page 51)	Chickpea and Vegetable Curry (Page 70)	Almond and Date Energy Balls (Page 88)
7	Sweet Potato and Black Bean Breakfast Burrito (Page 15)	Watermelon and Feta Salad (Page 52)	Lemon Garlic Herb Tilapia (Page 71)	Guacamole and Whole Grain Tortilla Chips (Page 89)
8	Blueberry Almond Oatmeal (Page 16)	Lentil and Vegetable Salad (Page 53)	Quinoa and Black Bean Enchiladas (Page 72)	Cottage Cheese and Pineapple Cups (Page 90)
9	Veggie-Packed Breakfast Casserole (Page 17)	Citrus and Arugula Salad (Page 54)	Baked Chicken with Mediterranean Salsa (Page 73)	Spicy Roasted Nuts Mix (Page 91)
10	Whole Grain Banana Pancakes (Page 18)	Roasted Vegetable and Farro Salad (Page 55)	Spinach and Mushroom Stuffed Chicken (Page 74)	Greek Yogurt and Cucumber Dip (Page 92)

Days 11-20

Day	Breakfast	Lunch	Dinner	Snacks
11	Tomato and Basil Breakfast Quiche (Page 19)	Kale and Cranberry Salad (Page 56)	Spaghetti Squash with Turkey Bolognese (Page 75)	Apple Slices with Almond Butter (Page 93)
12	Peanut Butter Banana Smoothie Bowl (Page 20)	Caprese Salad with Whole Wheat Croutons (Page 57)	Tofu and Vegetable Skewers (Page 76)	Quinoa and Kale Patties (Page 94)
13	Egg and Vegetable Breakfast Muffins (Page 21)	Asian Edamame and Noodle Salad (Page 58)	Zucchini Noodles with Pesto Shrimp (Page 77)	Carrot and Hummus Bites (Page 95)
14	Oat Bran Blueberry Muffins (Page 22)	Pomegranate and Walnut Spinach Salad (Page 59)	Cabbage and Turkey Sauté (Page 78)	Berry and Yogurt Parfait Pops (Page 96)
15	Shakshuka with Chickpeas (Page 23)	Shrimp and Avocado Salad (Page 60)	Sweet Potato and Black Bean Quesadillas (Page 79)	Whole Grain Crackers with Smoked Salmon (Page 97)
16	Spinach and Mushroom Breakfast Quesadilla (Page 24)	Caesar Salad with Grilled Chicken (Page 61)	Mediterranean Stuffed Portobello Mushrooms (Page 80)	Avocado and Tomato Salsa with Whole Wheat Chips (Page 98)
17	Greek Yogurt and Berry Smoothie (Page 25)	Mango and Quinoa Salad (Page 62)	Chicken and Broccoli Quinoa Bowl (Page 81)	Trail Mix with Nuts and Dried Fruit (Page 99)
18	Almond Butter and Banana Sandwich (Page 26)	Broccoli and Almond Salad (Page 63)	Moroccan Lentil and Vegetable Tagine (Page 82)	Dark Chocolate and Berry Bark (Page 101)
19	Mediterranean Egg White Omelette (Page 9)	Greek Salad with Quinoa (Page 46)	Grilled Lemon Herb Chicken (Page 65)	Greek Yogurt and Honey Frozen Bites (Page 102)
20	Quinoa and Vegetable Breakfast Bowl (Page 10)	Avocado and Chickpea Salad (Page 47)	Baked Salmon with Dill Sauce (Page 66)	Lemon Blueberry Chia Seed Pudding (Page 103)

Days 21-30

Day	Breakfast	Lunch	Dinner	Snacks
21	Berry Chia Seed Pudding (Page 11)	Spinach and Strawberry Salad (Page 48)	Turkey and Quinoa Stuffed Peppers (Page 67)	Almond Flour Banana Muffins (Page 104)
22	Spinach and Feta Breakfast Wrap (Page 12)	Cucumber and Tomato Salad with Feta (Page 49)	Eggplant and Lentil Moussaka (Page 68)	Berry and Oat Crumble Bars (Page 105)
23	Smoked Salmon Avocado Toast (Page 13)	Tuna and White Bean Salad (Page 50)	Shrimp and Vegetable Stir-Fry (Page 69)	Chocolate Avocado Mousse (Page 106)
24	Greek Yogurt Parfait with Mixed Berries (Page 14)	Quinoa and Black Bean Salad (Page 51)	Chickpea and Vegetable Curry (Page 70)	Coconut and Mango Sorbet (Page 107)
25	Sweet Potato and Black Bean Breakfast Burrito (Page 15)	Watermelon and Feta Salad (Page 52)	Lemon Garlic Herb Tilapia (Page 71)	Pistachio and Date Energy Bites (Page 108)
26	Blueberry Almond Oatmeal (Page 16)	Lentil and Vegetable Salad (Page 53)	Quinoa and Black Bean Enchiladas (Page 72)	Orange and Walnut Quinoa Cookies (Page 109)
27	Veggie-Packed Breakfast Casserole (Page 17)	Citrus and Arugula Salad (Page 54)	Baked Chicken with Mediterranean Salsa (Page 73)	Cinnamon Baked Apples (Page 110)
28	Whole Grain Banana Pancakes (Page 18)	Roasted Vegetable and Farro Salad (Page 55)	Spinach and Mushroom Stuffed Chicken (Page 74)	Raspberry Almond Chia Seed Parfait (Page 111)
29	Tomato and Basil Breakfast Quiche (Page 19)	Kale and Cranberry Salad (Page 56)	Spaghetti Squash with Turkey Bolognese (Page 75)	Whole Wheat Chocolate Chip Cookies (Page 112)
30	Peanut Butter Banana Smoothie Bowl (Page 20)	Caprese Salad with Whole Wheat Croutons (Page 57)	Tofu and Vegetable Skewers (Page 76)	Vanilla Bean and Berry Popsicles (Page 113)

Chapter 3: Breakfast

<u>Mediterranean Egg White Omelette</u>

Prep Time: 10 minutes | **Cook Time:** 10 minutes | **Servings:** 2

Ingredients:

- 1 cup egg whites
- 1/4 cup diced tomatoes
- 1/4 cup chopped spinach
- 2 tablespoons chopped red onions
- 2 tablespoons sliced black olives
- 1 tablespoon crumbled feta cheese
- 1 teaspoon olive oil
- 1/2 teaspoon dried oregano
- Salt and pepper to taste

Instructions:

1. In a bowl, whisk together the egg whites, dried oregano, salt, and pepper until well combined.
2. Heat olive oil in a non-stick skillet over medium heat.
3. Add chopped red onions to the skillet and sauté until they become translucent.
4. Add diced tomatoes and sliced black olives to the skillet. Sauté for an additional 2 minutes.
5. Add chopped spinach to the skillet and cook until it wilts.
6. Pour the whisked egg whites evenly over the sautéed vegetables in the skillet.
7. Allow the omelette to cook undisturbed for a few minutes until the edges set.
8. Gently lift the edges with a spatula, allowing any uncooked egg to flow underneath.
9. Once the omelette is mostly set, sprinkle crumbled feta cheese over one half of the omelette.
10. Carefully fold the other half of the omelette over the cheese, creating a half-moon shape.
11. Cook for an additional 2-3 minutes until the cheese melts and the omelette is fully cooked.
12. Slide the Mediterranean Egg White Omelette onto a plate and serve immediately.

Nutritional Information (per serving):

- **Carbs:** 8g
- **Sodium:** 450mg
- **Phosphorus:** 150mg
- **Potassium:** 300mg
- **Protein:** 20g

Quinoa and Vegetable Breakfast Bowl
Prep Time: 15 minutes | **Cook Time:** 20 minutes | **Servings:** 4

Ingredients:

- 1 cup quinoa, rinsed
- 2 cups water
- 1 tablespoon olive oil
- 1 cup diced bell peppers (red and yellow)
- 1 cup cherry tomatoes, halved
- 1 cup chopped spinach

- 1/2 cup diced red onions
- 2 cloves garlic, minced
- 1 teaspoon dried thyme
- Salt and pepper to taste
- 4 poached eggs (optional)
- 1 avocado, sliced (for garnish)

Instructions:

1. In a medium saucepan, combine quinoa and water. Bring to a boil, then reduce heat to low, cover, and simmer for 15 minutes or until quinoa is cooked and water is absorbed.

2. While quinoa is cooking, heat olive oil in a large skillet over medium heat.

3. Add diced red onions to the skillet and sauté until they become translucent.

4. Add minced garlic to the skillet and sauté for an additional 30 seconds.

5. Stir in diced bell peppers and continue to sauté until they are tender-crisp.

6. Add halved cherry tomatoes and chopped spinach to the skillet. Sauté until spinach wilts.

7. Once quinoa is cooked, fluff it with a fork and add it to the skillet with the sautéed vegetables.

8. Sprinkle dried thyme over the mixture and season with salt and pepper to taste. Stir to combine.

9. If desired, poach eggs separately.

10. Divide the quinoa and vegetable mixture among serving bowls. Top each bowl with a poached egg (if using) and garnish with sliced avocado.

11. Serve the Quinoa and Vegetable Breakfast Bowl immediately.

Nutritional Information (per serving):

- **Carbs:** 35g
- **Sodium:** 200mg
- **Phosphorus:** 220mg
- **Potassium:** 650mg
- **Protein:** 12g

Berry Chia Seed Pudding

Prep Time: 10 minutes (plus chilling time) | **Cook Time:** 0 minutes | **Servings:** 4

Ingredients:

- 1 cup unsweetened almond milk
- 1 cup mixed berries (strawberries, blueberries, raspberries)
- 1/4 cup chia seeds
- 2 tablespoons honey or maple syrup
- 1 teaspoon vanilla extract

Instructions:

1. In a blender, combine almond milk, mixed berries, honey (or maple syrup), and vanilla extract. Blend until smooth.
2. In a mixing bowl, pour the blended berry mixture over chia seeds. Stir adequately to combine.
3. Cover the bowl and refrigerate for at least 4 hours or overnight, allowing the chia seeds to absorb the liquid and create a pudding-like consistency.
4. Before serving, stir the chia pudding to ensure an even texture.
5. Divide the Berry Chia Seed Pudding into four servings.
6. Garnish each serving with additional berries for freshness.

Nutritional Information (per serving):

- **Carbs:** 20g
- **Sodium:** 40mg
- **Phosphorus:** 150mg
- **Potassium:** 220mg
- **Protein:** 4g

Spinach and Feta Breakfast Wrap

Prep Time: 10 minutes | **Cook Time:** 5 minutes | **Servings:** 2

Ingredients:

- 4 large eggs
- 1 cup fresh spinach leaves
- 1/4 cup crumbled feta cheese
- 1/4 cup diced tomatoes
- 2 whole wheat tortillas
- 1 tablespoon olive oil
- Salt and pepper to taste

Instructions:

1. In a bowl, whisk the eggs until well beaten. Season with salt and pepper to taste.
2. Heat olive oil in a non-stick skillet over medium heat.
3. Add fresh spinach leaves to the skillet and sauté until wilted.
4. Pour the beaten eggs into the skillet with the sautéed spinach.
5. Cook the eggs, stirring occasionally, until they are just set.
6. Sprinkle crumbled feta cheese over the eggs and stir until the cheese is slightly melted.
7. Add diced tomatoes to the skillet and stir for an additional 1-2 minutes.
8. Warm the whole wheat tortillas in a separate pan or microwave.
9. Divide the spinach and feta egg mixture evenly between the two tortillas.
10. Fold the sides of each tortilla and roll them into wraps.
11. Serve the Spinach and Feta Breakfast Wrap immediately.

Nutritional Information (per serving):

- **Carbs:** 30g
- **Sodium:** 450mg
- **Phosphorus:** 220mg
- **Potassium:** 300mg
- **Protein:** 20g

Smoked Salmon Avocado Toast

Prep Time: 10 minutes | **Cook Time:** 5 minutes | **Servings:** 2

Ingredients:

- 2 slices whole grain bread
- 1 ripe avocado, sliced
- 4 oz smoked salmon
- 1 tablespoon capers
- 1 tablespoon red onion, thinly sliced
- 1 tablespoon fresh dill, chopped
- 1 tablespoon lemon juice
- Salt and pepper to taste

Instructions:

1. Toast the whole grain bread slices to your desired level of crispiness.
2. While the bread is toasting, slice the ripe avocado and drizzle the slices with lemon juice to prevent browning.
3. Once the toast is ready, place sliced avocado evenly on each slice.
4. Layer smoked salmon over the avocado slices.
5. Sprinkle capers, thinly sliced red onion, and fresh dill over the smoked salmon.
6. Season the Smoked Salmon Avocado Toast with salt and pepper to taste.
7. Serve immediately, and enjoy your heart-healthy breakfast.

Nutritional Information (per serving):

- **Carbs:** 30g
- **Sodium:** 600mg
- **Phosphorus:** 200mg
- **Potassium:** 500mg
- **Protein:** 20g

Greek Yogurt Parfait with Mixed Berries

Prep Time: 10 minutes | **Cook Time:** 0 minutes | **Servings:** 2

Ingredients:

- 2 cups non-fat Greek yogurt

- 1 cup mixed berries (strawberries, blueberries, raspberries)

- 1/4 cup granola

- 2 tablespoons honey

- 1/4 teaspoon vanilla extract

- Mint leaves for garnish (optional)

Instructions:

1. In a bowl, mix non-fat Greek yogurt with vanilla extract until well combined.

2. Wash and prepare the mixed berries. If strawberries are used, hull and slice them.

3. In serving glasses or bowls, layer the Greek yogurt with the mixed berries.

4. Sprinkle granola over each layer for added texture and crunch.

5. Drizzle honey over the parfait for sweetness.

6. Repeat the layering process until the glasses are filled, finishing with a layer of mixed berries on top.

7. Garnish with mint leaves if desired.

8. Serve the Greek Yogurt Parfait with Mixed Berries immediately.

Nutritional Information (per serving):

- **Carbs:** 40g

- **Sodium:** 70mg

- **Phosphorus:** 300mg

- **Potassium:** 400mg

- **Protein:** 20g

Sweet Potato and Black Bean Breakfast Burrito

Prep Time: 15 minutes | **Cook Time:** 20 minutes | **Servings:** 4

Ingredients:

- 2 medium sweet potatoes, peeled and diced
- 1 can (15 oz) black beans, drained and rinsed
- 1 cup diced bell peppers (red and green)
- 1/2 cup diced red onions
- 1 teaspoon olive oil
- 1 teaspoon ground cumin
- 1/2 teaspoon chili powder
- Salt and pepper to taste
- 4 whole wheat tortillas
- 4 large eggs (optional)
- Salsa and avocado slices for topping

Instructions:

1. Preheat the oven to 400°F (200°C).

2. Toss diced sweet potatoes with olive oil, ground cumin, chili powder, salt, and pepper.

3. Spread the seasoned sweet potatoes on a baking sheet in a single layer. Roast in the preheated oven for 15-20 minutes or until tender and slightly crispy.

4. In a skillet over medium heat, sauté diced red onions and bell peppers until they are softened.

5. Add black beans to the skillet with the sautéed vegetables. Stir and cook for an additional 3-4 minutes.

6. Once the sweet potatoes are roasted, add them to the skillet and mix adequately.

7. Warm whole wheat tortillas in a separate pan or microwave.

8. Optional: In the same skillet, cook eggs to your liking (scrambled, fried, or poached).

9. Divide the sweet potato and black bean mixture among the warm tortillas.

10. If desired, top each burrito with a cooked egg.

11. Roll the Sweet Potato and Black Bean Breakfast Burritos, folding in the sides to secure the filling.

12. Serve with salsa and avocado slices.

Nutritional Information (per serving):

- **Carbs:** 40g
- **Sodium:** 500mg
- **Phosphorus:** 250mg
- **Potassium:** 700mg
- **Protein:** 15g

Blueberry Almond Oatmeal

Prep Time: 5 minutes | **Cook Time:** 10 minutes | **Servings:** 2

Ingredients:

- 1 cup old-fashioned oats

- 2 cups unsweetened almond milk

- 1 cup fresh or frozen blueberries

- 2 tablespoons almonds, sliced

- 1 tablespoon honey

- 1/2 teaspoon vanilla extract

- Pinch of salt

Instructions:

1. In a saucepan, combine old-fashioned oats and unsweetened almond milk.

2. Add a pinch of salt to the oats and almond milk mixture.

3. Bring the mixture to a gentle boil over medium heat, stirring occasionally.

4. Reduce heat to low and simmer for about 5-7 minutes, or until the oats reach your desired consistency.

5. While the oats are cooking, toast sliced almonds in a dry skillet over medium heat until they are golden brown. Be cautious not to burn them.

6. Once the oats are cooked, stir in honey and vanilla extract. Adjust sweetness to taste.

7. Fold in fresh or frozen blueberries to the oatmeal. If using frozen blueberries, allow them to heat through for a couple of minutes.

8. Take out the Blueberry Almond Oatmeal from heat.

9. Serve the oatmeal in bowls, topped with toasted sliced almonds.

Nutritional Information (per serving):

- **Carbs:** 50g

- **Sodium:** 150mg

- **Phosphorus:** 300mg

- **Potassium:** 350mg

- **Protein:** 10g

<u>Veggie-Packed Breakfast Casserole</u>

Prep Time: 20 minutes | **Cook Time:** 40 minutes | **Servings:** 6

Ingredients:

- 8 large eggs
- 1 cup skim milk
- 2 cups diced sweet potatoes
- 1 cup broccoli florets, chopped
- 1/2 cup red bell pepper, diced
- 1/2 cup yellow bell pepper, diced
- 1/2 cup cherry tomatoes, halved
- 1 cup baby spinach, chopped
- 1 cup reduced-fat shredded cheddar cheese
- 1 teaspoon olive oil
- 1 teaspoon garlic powder
- 1 teaspoon onion powder
- Salt and pepper to taste

Instructions:

1. Preheat the oven to 375°F (190°C).

2. In a skillet, heat olive oil over medium heat. Sauté diced sweet potatoes until they are slightly softened.

3. Add diced red and yellow bell peppers to the skillet with the sweet potatoes. Sauté until the vegetables are tender.

4. In a bowl, whisk together eggs, skim milk, garlic powder, onion powder, salt, and pepper.

5. In a greased baking dish, layer the sautéed sweet potatoes and peppers, broccoli florets, halved cherry tomatoes, and chopped baby spinach.

6. Pour the egg mixture evenly over the layered vegetables in the baking dish.

7. Sprinkle reduced-fat shredded cheddar cheese over the top.

8. Bake the Veggie-Packed Breakfast Casserole in the preheated oven for 35-40 minutes or until the eggs are set and the top is golden brown.

9. Allow the casserole to cool slightly before slicing and serving.

Nutritional Information (per serving):

- **Carbs:** 20g
- **Sodium:** 400mg
- **Phosphorus:** 250mg
- **Potassium:** 450mg
- **Protein:** 15g

Whole Grain Banana Pancakes

Prep Time: 10 minutes | **Cook Time:** 10 minutes | **Servings:** 4

Ingredients:

- 1 cup whole wheat flour
- 1/2 cup old-fashioned oats
- 2 teaspoons baking powder
- 1/2 teaspoon cinnamon
- 1/4 teaspoon salt
- 1 cup skim milk

- 2 ripe bananas, mashed
- 1 large egg
- 1 tablespoon honey
- 1 teaspoon vanilla extract
- Cooking spray or oil for the pan

Instructions:

1. In a large bowl, whisk together whole wheat flour, old-fashioned oats, baking powder, cinnamon, and salt.

2. In a separate bowl, combine skim milk, mashed bananas, egg, honey, and vanilla extract. Mix adequately.

3. Pour the wet ingredients into the dry ingredients and stir until just combined. Do not overmix; a few lumps are okay.

4. Preheat a non-stick skillet or griddle over medium heat. Lightly coat with cooking spray or a small amount of oil.

5. Pour 1/4 cup of batter onto the skillet for each pancake. Cook until bubbles form on the surface, then flip and cook the other side until golden brown.

6. Repeat until all the batter is used, adjusting the heat if necessary to prevent burning.

7. Serve the Whole Grain Banana Pancakes warm, topped with additional banana slices or berries if desired.

Nutritional Information (per serving):

- **Carbs:** 40g
- **Sodium:** 350mg
- **Phosphorus:** 200mg
- **Potassium:** 450mg
- **Protein:** 10g

Tomato and Basil Breakfast Quiche

Prep Time: 15 minutes | **Cook Time:** 40 minutes | **Servings:** 6

Ingredients:

- 1 pre-made whole wheat pie crust
- 1 cup cherry tomatoes, halved
- 1 cup fresh spinach, chopped
- 1/2 cup red bell pepper, diced
- 1/4 cup fresh basil, chopped
- 1 cup skim milk
- 4 large eggs
- 1 cup reduced-fat feta cheese, crumbled
- 1 teaspoon olive oil
- Salt and pepper to taste

Instructions:

1. Preheat the oven to 375°F (190°C).
2. In a skillet, heat olive oil over medium heat. Add diced red bell pepper and sauté until softened.
3. Roll out the whole wheat pie crust and press it into a pie dish.
4. In a bowl, whisk together skim milk, eggs, salt, and pepper until well combined.
5. Sprinkle crumbled reduced-fat feta cheese over the pie crust.
6. Spread sautéed red bell pepper evenly over the cheese.
7. Add chopped fresh spinach and halved cherry tomatoes to the pie dish, distributing them evenly.
8. Pour the egg mixture over the vegetables and cheese in the pie dish.
9. Sprinkle chopped fresh basil over the top.
10. Bake the Tomato and Basil Breakfast Quiche in the preheated oven for 35-40 minutes or until the center is set and the top is golden brown.
11. Allow the quiche to cool slightly before slicing and serving.

Nutritional Information (per serving):

- **Carbs:** 20g
- **Sodium:** 400mg
- **Phosphorus:** 250mg
- **Potassium:** 350mg
- **Protein:** 15g

Peanut Butter Banana Smoothie Bowl

Prep Time: 5 minutes | **Cook Time:** 0 minutes | **Servings:** 2

Ingredients:

- 2 ripe bananas, sliced and frozen
- 1/2 cup non-fat Greek yogurt
- 1/4 cup skim milk
- 2 tablespoons peanut butter
- 1 tablespoon honey
- 1/4 cup granola
- 2 tablespoons unsalted peanuts, chopped
- 1 tablespoon chia seeds
- Sliced strawberries and banana for topping

Instructions:

1. In a blender, combine frozen banana slices, non-fat Greek yogurt, skim milk, peanut butter, and honey.
2. Blend the ingredients until smooth and creamy, adjusting the consistency with more milk if needed.
3. Pour the Peanut Butter Banana Smoothie into bowls.
4. Top the smoothie bowls with granola, chopped unsalted peanuts, chia seeds, and sliced strawberries and bananas.
5. Serve the smoothie bowls immediately.

Nutritional Information (per serving):

- **Carbs:** 40g
- **Sodium:** 80mg
- **Phosphorus:** 220mg
- **Potassium:** 550mg
- **Protein:** 10g

Egg and Vegetable Breakfast Muffins

Prep Time: 15 minutes | **Cook Time:** 20 minutes | **Servings:** 6

Ingredients:

- 6 large eggs
- 1/2 cup skim milk
- 1 cup cherry tomatoes, diced
- 1/2 cup red bell pepper, diced
- 1/2 cup green bell pepper, diced
- 1/2 cup red onion, diced
- 1/2 cup spinach, chopped
- 1/4 cup reduced-fat feta cheese, crumbled
- 1 teaspoon olive oil
- 1/2 teaspoon garlic powder
- Salt and pepper to taste
- Cooking spray

Instructions:

1. Preheat the oven to 375°F (190°C). Grease a muffin tin with cooking spray.

2. In a skillet, heat olive oil over medium heat. Sauté diced red and green bell peppers and red onions until softened.

3. In a bowl, whisk together eggs, skim milk, garlic powder, salt, and pepper until well combined.

4. Distribute the sautéed vegetables evenly among the muffin tin cups.

5. Pour the egg mixture over the vegetables in each muffin cup.

6. Add diced cherry tomatoes and chopped spinach to each muffin cup, distributing them evenly.

7. Sprinkle crumbled reduced-fat feta cheese over the top.

8. Bake the Egg and Vegetable Breakfast Muffins in the preheated oven for 15-20 minutes or until the eggs are set and the tops are golden brown.

9. Allow the muffins to cool slightly before removing them from the tin.

10. Serve the muffins warm.

Nutritional Information (per serving):

- **Carbs:** 5g
- **Sodium:** 300mg
- **Phosphorus:** 150mg
- **Potassium:** 250mg
- **Protein:** 10g

Oat Bran Blueberry Muffins

Prep Time: 15 minutes | **Cook Time:** 20 minutes | **Servings:** 12

Ingredients:

- 1 cup oat bran
- 1 cup whole wheat flour
- 1/2 cup brown sugar
- 1 teaspoon baking powder
- 1/2 teaspoon baking soda
- 1/2 teaspoon cinnamon
- 1/4 teaspoon salt
- 1 cup skim milk
- 1/4 cup unsweetened applesauce
- 2 tablespoons olive oil
- 1 large egg
- 1 teaspoon vanilla extract
- 1 cup blueberries (fresh or frozen)

Instructions:

1. Preheat the oven to 375°F (190°C). Line a muffin tin with paper liners.
2. In a large bowl, combine oat bran, whole wheat flour, brown sugar, baking powder, baking soda, cinnamon, and salt.
3. In a separate bowl, whisk together skim milk, unsweetened applesauce, olive oil, egg, and vanilla extract.
4. Pour the wet ingredients into the dry ingredients and stir until just combined.
5. Gently fold in blueberries to the batter.
6. Spoon the batter into the muffin tin, filling each cup about two-thirds full.
7. Bake the Oat Bran Blueberry Muffins in the preheated oven for 18-20 minutes or until a toothpick inserted into the center comes out clean.
8. Allow the muffins to cool in the tin for a few minutes before transferring them to a wire rack to cool completely.
9. Serve the muffins at room temperature.

Nutritional Information (per serving):

- **Carbs:** 25g
- **Sodium:** 150mg
- **Phosphorus:** 100mg
- **Potassium:** 200mg
- **Protein:** 3g

Shakshuka with Chickpeas

Prep Time: 10 minutes | **Cook Time:** 25 minutes | **Servings:** 4

Ingredients:

- 2 tablespoons olive oil
- 1 large onion, finely chopped
- 1 red bell pepper, diced
- 3 cloves garlic, minced
- 1 teaspoon ground cumin
- 1 teaspoon ground coriander
- 1 teaspoon smoked paprika
- 1/2 teaspoon cayenne pepper (optional)
- 1 can (28 oz) crushed tomatoes
- 1 can (15 oz) chickpeas, drained and rinsed
- 4-6 large eggs
- Salt and pepper to taste
- Fresh cilantro or parsley for garnish

Instructions:

1. In a large skillet, heat olive oil over medium heat.

2. Add finely chopped onion and diced red bell pepper to the skillet. Sauté until vegetables are softened.

3. Stir in minced garlic, ground cumin, ground coriander, smoked paprika, and cayenne pepper (if using). Sauté for an additional 1-2 minutes until the spices are fragrant.

4. Pour in the can of crushed tomatoes and add drained and rinsed chickpeas. Stir to combine.

5. Simmer the mixture over medium-low heat for 10-15 minutes, allowing the flavors to meld.

6. Create small wells in the tomato-chickpea mixture and carefully crack eggs into each well.

7. Cover the skillet and cook for an additional 8-10 minutes, or until the eggs are cooked to your liking.

8. Season the Shakshuka with Chickpeas with salt and pepper to taste.

9. Garnish with fresh cilantro or parsley.

10. Serve the Shakshuka with Chickpeas hot, directly from the skillet.

Nutritional Information (per serving):

- **Carbs:** 25g
- **Sodium:** 600mg
- **Phosphorus:** 150mg
- **Potassium:** 550mg
- **Protein:** 15g

Spinach and Mushroom Breakfast Quesadilla

Prep Time: 10 minutes | **Cook Time:** 10 minutes | **Servings:** 2

Ingredients:

- 4 whole wheat tortillas
- 1 cup fresh spinach leaves
- 1 cup cremini mushrooms, sliced
- 1/2 cup red onion, thinly sliced
- 1/2 cup reduced-fat shredded cheddar cheese

- 4 large eggs
- 1 tablespoon olive oil
- Salt and pepper to taste
- Salsa for serving (optional)

Instructions:

1. In a skillet, heat olive oil over medium heat.
2. Add thinly sliced red onion to the skillet. Sauté until softened.
3. Add sliced cremini mushrooms to the skillet. Sauté until the mushrooms are browned.
4. Push the vegetables to the side of the skillet and crack the eggs into the empty side. Scramble the eggs until they are cooked through.
5. Mix the scrambled eggs with the sautéed mushrooms and onions in the skillet.
6. Season the egg and vegetable mixture with salt and pepper to taste.
7. Place one whole wheat tortilla in the skillet. Spoon half of the egg and vegetable mixture onto half of the tortilla.
8. Add a handful of fresh spinach leaves on top of the egg mixture.
9. Sprinkle half of the reduced-fat shredded cheddar cheese over the spinach.
10. Fold the tortilla in half to cover the filling. Press down gently with a spatula.
11. Cook the Spinach and Mushroom Breakfast Quesadilla for 2-3 minutes on each side, or until the tortilla is golden brown and the cheese is melted.
12. Repeat the process with the remaining ingredients to make the second quesadilla.
13. Serve the quesadillas hot, with salsa on the side if desired.

Nutritional Information (per serving):

- **Carbs:** 35g
- **Sodium:** 350mg
- **Phosphorus:** 250mg
- **Potassium:** 300mg
- **Protein:** 20g

Greek Yogurt and Berry Smoothie

Prep Time: 5 minutes | **Cook Time:** 0 minutes | **Servings:** 2

Ingredients:

- 1 cup non-fat Greek yogurt
- 1/2 cup skim milk
- 1 cup mixed berries (strawberries, blueberries, raspberries)
- 1 medium banana, sliced
- 1 tablespoon honey
- 1/4 cup rolled oats
- 1/2 teaspoon vanilla extract
- Ice cubes (optional)

Instructions:

1. In a blender, combine non-fat Greek yogurt, skim milk, mixed berries, sliced banana, honey, rolled oats, and vanilla extract.
2. If a colder and thicker consistency is desired, add ice cubes to the blender.
3. Blend the ingredients until smooth and well combined.
4. Pour the Greek Yogurt and Berry Smoothie into glasses.
5. Garnish with additional berries or a drizzle of honey if desired.
6. Serve the smoothie immediately.

Nutritional Information (per serving):

- **Carbs:** 40g
- **Sodium:** 90mg
- **Phosphorus:** 250mg
- **Potassium:** 500mg
- **Protein:** 15g

Almond Butter and Banana Sandwich

Prep Time: 5 minutes | **Cook Time:** 0 minutes | **Servings:** 2

Ingredients:

- 4 slices whole grain bread
- 4 tablespoons almond butter
- 2 medium bananas, sliced
- 1 tablespoon honey
- 1/2 teaspoon cinnamon

Instructions:

1. Lay out the slices of whole grain bread on a clean surface.
2. Spread 2 tablespoons of almond butter evenly on two slices of the bread.
3. Arrange sliced bananas over the almond butter on each of the two slices.
4. Drizzle honey evenly over the banana slices.
5. Sprinkle a pinch of cinnamon over the banana slices for added flavor.
6. Place the remaining slices of whole grain bread on top to form sandwiches.
7. Press down gently to secure the sandwiches.
8. Optionally, cut the sandwiches in half for easier handling.
9. Serve the Almond Butter and Banana Sandwiches immediately.

Nutritional Information (per serving):

- **Carbs:** 50g
- **Sodium:** 200mg
- **Phosphorus:** 250mg
- **Potassium:** 450mg
- **Protein:** 10g

Chapter 4: Soups and Stews

Lentil and Vegetable Soup

Prep Time: 15 minutes | **Cook Time:** 45 minutes | **Number of Servings:** 6

Ingredients:

- 1 cup dried green lentils, rinsed and drained
- 1 large onion, diced
- 3 carrots, sliced
- 3 celery stalks, diced
- 3 cloves garlic, minced
- 1 can (14 oz) diced tomatoes, undrained
- 6 cups low-sodium vegetable broth
- 1 teaspoon dried thyme
- 1 teaspoon dried rosemary
- 1/2 teaspoon ground black pepper
- 2 cups chopped kale
- 1 tablespoon olive oil
- Salt to taste

Instructions:

1. In a large pot, heat olive oil over medium heat. Add diced onion, sliced carrots, diced celery, and minced garlic. Sauté until vegetables are tender.

2. Add rinsed lentils, diced tomatoes (with their juice), vegetable broth, thyme, rosemary, and black pepper to the pot. Stir adequately.

3. Bring the soup to a boil, then reduce the heat to low, cover, and simmer for 30-35 minutes or until lentils are tender.

4. Add chopped kale to the pot and cook for an additional 5-7 minutes until the kale is wilted.

5. Season the soup with salt to taste. Adjust the seasoning if necessary.

6. Serve the lentil and vegetable soup hot. Enjoy your heart-healthy DASH diet meal!

Nutritional Information (Per Serving):

- **Carbs:** 40g
- **Sodium:** 350mg
- **Phosphorus:** 180mg
- **Potassium:** 600mg
- **Protein:** 12g

<u>**Chicken and Quinoa Soup**</u>

Prep Time: 20 minutes | **Cook Time:** 30 minutes | **Number of Servings:** 4

Ingredients:

- 1 cup quinoa, rinsed and drained
- 1 pound boneless, skinless chicken breasts, diced
- 1 tablespoon olive oil
- 1 large onion, finely chopped
- 3 carrots, sliced
- 3 celery stalks, diced
- 3 cloves garlic, minced
- 6 cups low-sodium chicken broth
- 1 teaspoon dried thyme
- 1 teaspoon dried rosemary
- 1/2 teaspoon ground black pepper
- 1 cup green beans, trimmed and cut into 1-inch pieces
- 1 cup spinach, chopped
- Salt to taste

Instructions:

1. In a large pot, heat olive oil over medium heat. Add finely chopped onion, sliced carrots, diced celery, and minced garlic. Sauté until vegetables are softened.

2. Add diced chicken to the pot and cook until browned on all sides.

3. Pour in the chicken broth, add rinsed quinoa, thyme, rosemary, and black pepper. Stir adequately.

4. Bring the soup to a boil, then reduce the heat to low, cover, and simmer for 20 minutes or until quinoa is cooked.

5. Add green beans to the pot and cook for an additional 5-7 minutes until the beans are tender.

6. Stir in chopped spinach and cook until wilted.

7. Season the soup with salt to taste. Adjust the seasoning if needed.

8. Serve the chicken and quinoa soup hot. Enjoy your heart-healthy DASH diet meal!

Nutritional Information (Per Serving):

- **Carbs:** 35g
- **Sodium:** 400mg
- **Phosphorus:** 220mg
- **Potassium:** 500mg
- **Protein:** 25g

Spicy Black Bean Chili

Prep Time: 15 minutes | **Cook Time:** 40 minutes | **Number of Servings:** 8

Ingredients:

- 2 cans (15 oz each) black beans, drained and rinsed
- 1 pound lean ground turkey
- 1 tablespoon olive oil
- 1 large onion, diced
- 3 bell peppers (assorted colors), diced
- 4 cloves garlic, minced
- 1 can (28 oz) crushed tomatoes
- 2 cups low-sodium vegetable broth
- 2 tablespoons chili powder
- 1 tablespoon ground cumin
- 1 teaspoon smoked paprika
- 1/2 teaspoon cayenne pepper (adjust to taste)
- Salt to taste
- Chopped fresh cilantro for garnish (optional)
- Plain Greek yogurt for serving (optional)

Instructions:

1. In a large pot, heat olive oil over medium heat. Add diced onion, diced bell peppers, and minced garlic. Sauté until vegetables are tender.

2. Add ground turkey to the pot and cook until browned.

3. Stir in chili powder, ground cumin, smoked paprika, and cayenne pepper. Cook for 2-3 minutes to allow the spices to toast.

4. Pour in crushed tomatoes and vegetable broth. Add drained and rinsed black beans. Stir adequately.

5. Bring the chili to a boil, then reduce the heat to low, cover, and simmer for 30 minutes, stirring occasionally.

6. Season the chili with salt to taste. Adjust the seasoning if necessary.

7. Serve the spicy black bean chili hot, garnished with chopped cilantro and a dollop of plain Greek yogurt if desired. Enjoy your heart-healthy DASH diet meal!

Nutritional Information (Per Serving):

- **Carbs:** 25g
- **Sodium:** 300mg
- **Phosphorus:** 200mg
- **Potassium:** 400mg
- **Protein:** 20g

Tomato Basil White Bean Soup

Prep Time: 15 minutes | **Cook Time:** 25 minutes | **Number of Servings:** 6

Ingredients:

- 2 cans (15 oz each) white beans, drained and rinsed
- 1 tablespoon olive oil
- 1 large onion, finely chopped
- 3 cloves garlic, minced
- 2 cans (14 oz each) diced tomatoes, undrained
- 4 cups low-sodium vegetable broth
- 1 teaspoon dried oregano
- 1 teaspoon dried basil
- 1/2 teaspoon black pepper
- 1/4 teaspoon red pepper flakes (optional)
- Salt to taste
- 1/4 cup fresh basil, thinly sliced, for garnish
- Grated Parmesan cheese for serving (optional)

Instructions:

1. In a large pot, heat olive oil over medium heat. Add finely chopped onion and minced garlic. Sauté until the onion is translucent.

2. Add diced tomatoes (with their juice) to the pot, along with drained and rinsed white beans. Stir adequately.

3. Pour in vegetable broth and add dried oregano, dried basil, black pepper, and red pepper flakes. Bring the soup to a simmer.

4. Allow the soup to simmer for 15-20 minutes, allowing the flavors to meld together.

5. Season the soup with salt to taste. Adjust the seasoning if necessary.

6. Ladle the tomato basil white bean soup into bowls and garnish with thinly sliced fresh basil.

7. Optionally, serve with a sprinkle of grated Parmesan cheese on top.

8. Enjoy your heart-healthy DASH diet meal!

Nutritional Information (Per Serving):

- **Carbs:** 30g
- **Sodium:** 350mg
- **Phosphorus:** 180mg
- **Potassium:** 400mg
- **Protein:** 10g

Turkey and Vegetable Stew

Prep Time: 20 minutes | **Cook Time:** 40 minutes | **Number of Servings:** 6

Ingredients:

- 1.5 pounds lean ground turkey
- 1 tablespoon olive oil
- 1 large onion, diced
- 3 carrots, sliced
- 3 celery stalks, diced
- 3 cloves garlic, minced
- 1 can (14 oz) diced tomatoes, undrained
- 4 cups low-sodium chicken broth
- 1 teaspoon dried thyme
- 1 teaspoon dried rosemary
- 1/2 teaspoon black pepper
- 2 cups green beans, trimmed and cut into 1-inch pieces
- 2 cups sweet potatoes, peeled and diced
- Salt to taste

Instructions:

1. In a large pot, heat olive oil over medium heat. Add diced onion, sliced carrots, diced celery, and minced garlic. Sauté until vegetables are tender.

2. Add ground turkey to the pot and cook until browned.

3. Stir in diced tomatoes (with their juice), chicken broth, thyme, rosemary, and black pepper. Bring the stew to a boil, then reduce the heat to low, cover, and simmer for 25-30 minutes.

4. Add green beans and diced sweet potatoes to the pot. Continue to simmer for an additional 15-20 minutes or until the vegetables are fork-tender.

5. Season the stew with salt to taste. Adjust the seasoning if necessary.

6. Serve the turkey and vegetable stew hot. Enjoy your heart-healthy DASH diet meal!

Nutritional Information (Per Serving):

- **Carbs:** 30g
- **Sodium:** 400mg
- **Phosphorus:** 250mg
- **Potassium:** 600mg
- **Protein:** 25g

Lemon Chicken and Orzo Soup

Prep Time: 15 minutes | **Cook Time:** 25 minutes | **Number of Servings:** 4

Ingredients:

- 1 pound boneless, skinless chicken breasts, diced
- 1 tablespoon olive oil
- 1 large onion, finely chopped
- 3 carrots, sliced
- 3 celery stalks, diced
- 3 cloves garlic, minced
- 6 cups low-sodium chicken broth
- 1 cup orzo pasta
- 2 teaspoons dried thyme
- 2 tablespoons fresh lemon juice
- Zest of 1 lemon
- Salt and black pepper to taste
- 1/4 cup fresh parsley, chopped, for garnish

Instructions:

1. In a large pot, heat olive oil over medium heat. Add finely chopped onion, sliced carrots, diced celery, and minced garlic. Sauté until vegetables are tender.
2. Add diced chicken to the pot and cook until browned.
3. Pour in chicken broth and bring the soup to a simmer. Add orzo pasta and dried thyme. Cook until the orzo is tender, following the package instructions.
4. Stir in fresh lemon juice and lemon zest. Season the soup with salt and black pepper to taste.
5. Allow the soup to simmer for an additional 5 minutes to let the flavors meld together.
6. Ladle the lemon chicken and orzo soup into bowls and garnish with chopped fresh parsley.
7. Serve the soup hot. Enjoy your heart-healthy DASH diet meal!

Nutritional Information (Per Serving):

- **Carbs:** 40g
- **Sodium:** 350mg
- **Phosphorus:** 200mg
- **Potassium:** 400mg
- **Protein:** 25g

Minestrone Soup with Whole Wheat Pasta

Prep Time: 20 minutes | **Cook Time:** 30 minutes | **Number of Servings:** 6

Ingredients:

- 1 cup whole wheat pasta, uncooked
- 1 tablespoon olive oil
- 1 large onion, finely chopped
- 3 carrots, sliced
- 3 celery stalks, diced
- 3 cloves garlic, minced
- 1 can (14 oz) diced tomatoes, undrained
- 6 cups low-sodium vegetable broth
- 1 zucchini, diced
- 1 cup green beans, trimmed and cut into 1-inch pieces
- 1 can (15 oz) kidney beans, drained and rinsed
- 1 teaspoon dried oregano
- 1 teaspoon dried basil
- 1/2 teaspoon black pepper
- Salt to taste
- 1/4 cup fresh parsley, chopped, for garnish
- Grated Parmesan cheese for serving (optional)

Instructions:

1. Cook the whole wheat pasta according to the package instructions. Drain and set aside.
2. In a large pot, heat olive oil over medium heat. Add finely chopped onion, sliced carrots, diced celery, and minced garlic. Sauté until vegetables are tender.
3. Add diced tomatoes (with their juice) to the pot, along with low-sodium vegetable broth, diced zucchini, green beans, and drained kidney beans. Stir adequately.
4. Season the soup with dried oregano, dried basil, black pepper, and salt to taste. Bring the soup to a simmer.
5. Simmer the soup for 20-25 minutes, allowing the flavors to meld together.
6. Add the cooked whole wheat pasta to the pot and stir until well combined.
7. Ladle the minestrone soup into bowls, garnish with chopped fresh parsley, and optionally serve with grated Parmesan cheese on top.
8. Enjoy your heart-healthy DASH diet meal!

Nutritional Information (Per Serving):

- **Carbs:** 35g
- **Sodium:** 400mg
- **Phosphorus:** 250mg
- **Potassium:** 600mg
- **Protein:** 12g

<u>Sweet Potato and Kale Soup</u>

Prep Time: 20 minutes | **Cook Time:** 30 minutes | **Number of Servings:** 4

Ingredients:

- 2 large sweet potatoes, peeled and diced
- 1 tablespoon olive oil
- 1 large onion, finely chopped
- 3 cloves garlic, minced
- 6 cups low-sodium vegetable broth
- 4 cups kale, chopped
- 1 teaspoon dried thyme
- 1/2 teaspoon ground cumin
- 1/2 teaspoon paprika
- 1/4 teaspoon black pepper
- Salt to taste
- 1 can (15 oz) cannellini beans, drained and rinsed
- 1 tablespoon apple cider vinegar
- 1/4 cup fresh cilantro, chopped, for garnish

Instructions:

1. In a large pot, heat olive oil over medium heat. Add finely chopped onion and minced garlic. Sauté until the onion is translucent.

2. Add diced sweet potatoes to the pot and cook for 5 minutes, stirring occasionally.

3. Pour in low-sodium vegetable broth, add chopped kale, dried thyme, ground cumin, paprika, black pepper, and salt to taste. Stir adequately.

4. Bring the soup to a boil, then reduce the heat to low, cover, and simmer for 15-20 minutes or until sweet potatoes are tender.

5. Add drained and rinsed cannellini beans to the pot and cook for an additional 5 minutes.

6. Stir in apple cider vinegar to brighten the flavors. Adjust salt and pepper if needed.

7. Serve the sweet potato and kale soup hot, garnished with fresh cilantro.

8. Enjoy your heart-healthy DASH diet meal!

Nutritional Information (Per Serving):

- **Carbs:** 35g
- **Sodium:** 400mg
- **Phosphorus:** 200mg
- **Potassium:** 800mg
- **Protein:** 10g

Moroccan Chickpea Stew

Prep Time: 15 minutes | **Cook Time:** 40 minutes | **Number of Servings:** 6

Ingredients:

- 2 tablespoons olive oil
- 1 large onion, finely chopped
- 3 cloves garlic, minced
- 1 teaspoon ground cumin
- 1 teaspoon ground coriander
- 1/2 teaspoon ground cinnamon
- 1/2 teaspoon paprika
- 1/4 teaspoon cayenne pepper (adjust to taste)
- 1 can (14 oz) diced tomatoes, undrained
- 4 cups low-sodium vegetable broth
- 2 sweet potatoes, peeled and diced
- 3 carrots, sliced
- 1 cup dried red lentils, rinsed and drained
- 2 cans (15 oz each) chickpeas, drained and rinsed
- Salt and black pepper to taste
- 1/4 cup fresh cilantro, chopped, for garnish

Instructions:

1. In a large pot, heat olive oil over medium heat. Add finely chopped onion and minced garlic. Sauté until the onion is translucent.

2. Add ground cumin, ground coriander, ground cinnamon, paprika, and cayenne pepper to the pot. Cook for 2-3 minutes to toast the spices.

3. Pour in diced tomatoes (with their juice) and low-sodium vegetable broth. Stir adequately.

4. Add diced sweet potatoes, sliced carrots, and rinsed red lentils to the pot. Bring the stew to a simmer and cook for 20-25 minutes or until the vegetables and lentils are tender.

5. Stir in drained and rinsed chickpeas. Cook for an additional 10 minutes to heat through.

6. Season the stew with salt and black pepper to taste. Adjust the seasoning if necessary.

7. Serve the Moroccan chickpea stew hot, garnished with chopped fresh cilantro.

8. Enjoy your heart-healthy DASH diet meal!

Nutritional Information (Per Serving):

- **Carbs:** 45g
- **Sodium:** 400mg
- **Phosphorus:** 250mg
- **Potassium:** 800mg
- **Protein:** 15g

Spinach and Lentil Soup

Prep Time: 15 minutes | **Cook Time:** 40 minutes | **Number of Servings:** 6

Ingredients:

- 1 cup dried green lentils, rinsed and drained
- 1 tablespoon olive oil
- 1 large onion, finely chopped
- 3 carrots, sliced
- 3 celery stalks, diced
- 3 cloves garlic, minced
- 1 teaspoon ground cumin
- 1 teaspoon ground coriander
- 1/2 teaspoon smoked paprika
- 6 cups low-sodium vegetable broth
- 1 can (14 oz) diced tomatoes, undrained
- 4 cups fresh spinach, chopped
- Salt and black pepper to taste
- 1 lemon, sliced, for garnish
- 1/4 cup fresh parsley, chopped, for garnish

Instructions:

1. In a large pot, heat olive oil over medium heat. Add finely chopped onion, sliced carrots, diced celery, and minced garlic. Sauté until vegetables are tender.

2. Add ground cumin, ground coriander, and smoked paprika to the pot. Cook for 2-3 minutes to enhance the flavors.

3. Pour in low-sodium vegetable broth and add rinsed green lentils. Stir adequately.

4. Bring the soup to a boil, then reduce the heat to low, cover, and simmer for 25-30 minutes or until lentils are tender.

5. Add diced tomatoes (with their juice) to the pot, followed by chopped fresh spinach. Cook for an additional 5-7 minutes until the spinach is wilted.

6. Season the soup with salt and black pepper to taste. Adjust the seasoning if necessary.

7. Serve the spinach and lentil soup hot, garnished with slices of lemon and chopped fresh parsley.

8. Enjoy your heart-healthy DASH diet meal!

Nutritional Information (Per Serving):

- **Carbs:** 30g
- **Sodium:** 400mg
- **Phosphorus:** 200mg
- **Potassium:** 600mg
- **Protein:** 15g

Zucchini and Red Lentil Soup

Prep Time: 15 minutes | **Cook Time:** 35 minutes | **Number of Servings:** 4

Ingredients:

- 1 cup red lentils, rinsed and drained
- 1 tablespoon olive oil
- 1 large onion, finely chopped
- 3 cloves garlic, minced
- 4 zucchinis, diced
- 3 carrots, sliced
- 6 cups low-sodium vegetable broth
- 1 teaspoon ground cumin
- 1 teaspoon ground coriander
- 1/2 teaspoon turmeric
- 1/4 teaspoon cayenne pepper (adjust to taste)
- Salt and black pepper to taste
- 1 lemon, juiced
- 1/4 cup fresh cilantro, chopped, for garnish

Instructions:

1. In a large pot, heat olive oil over medium heat. Add finely chopped onion and minced garlic. Sauté until the onion is translucent.

2. Add diced zucchinis and sliced carrots to the pot. Cook for 5 minutes, stirring occasionally.

3. Pour in low-sodium vegetable broth and add rinsed red lentils. Stir adequately.

4. Season the soup with ground cumin, ground coriander, turmeric, cayenne pepper, salt, and black pepper. Bring the soup to a boil, then reduce the heat to low, cover, and simmer for 25-30 minutes or until lentils are tender.

5. Using an immersion blender, blend a portion of the soup to create a creamy texture while leaving some chunks for added texture.

6. Stir in freshly squeezed lemon juice. Adjust salt and pepper if needed.

7. Serve the zucchini and red lentil soup hot, garnished with chopped fresh cilantro.

8. Enjoy your heart-healthy DASH diet meal!

Nutritional Information (Per Serving):

- **Carbs:** 40g
- **Sodium:** 400mg
- **Phosphorus:** 250mg
- **Potassium:** 700mg
- **Protein:** 15g

<u>Mushroom Barley Soup</u>

Prep Time: 20 minutes | **Cook Time:** 45 minutes | **Number of Servings:** 6

Ingredients:

- 1 cup pearled barley
- 1 tablespoon olive oil
- 1 large onion, finely chopped
- 3 carrots, sliced
- 3 celery stalks, diced
- 3 cloves garlic, minced
- 1 pound mushrooms, sliced
- 8 cups low-sodium vegetable broth
- 2 teaspoons dried thyme
- 1 teaspoon dried rosemary
- 1/2 teaspoon black pepper
- Salt to taste
- 1/4 cup fresh parsley, chopped, for garnish

Instructions:

1. Rinse pearled barley under cold water and set aside.

2. In a large pot, heat olive oil over medium heat. Add finely chopped onion, sliced carrots, diced celery, and minced garlic. Sauté until vegetables are tender.

3. Add sliced mushrooms to the pot and cook for an additional 5 minutes.

4. Pour in low-sodium vegetable broth and add rinsed pearled barley. Stir adequately.

5. Season the soup with dried thyme, dried rosemary, black pepper, and salt to taste. Bring the soup to a boil, then reduce the heat to low, cover, and simmer for 35-40 minutes or until the barley is tender.

6. Adjust the seasoning if necessary.

7. Serve the mushroom barley soup hot, garnished with chopped fresh parsley.

8. Enjoy your heart-healthy DASH diet meal!

Nutritional Information (Per Serving):

- **Carbs:** 40g
- **Sodium:** 400mg
- **Phosphorus:** 200mg
- **Potassium:** 600mg
- **Protein:** 10g

Cabbage and White Bean Stew

Prep Time: 20 minutes | **Cook Time:** 35 minutes | **Number of Servings:** 4

Ingredients:

- 1 tablespoon olive oil
- 1 large onion, finely chopped
- 3 cloves garlic, minced
- 1 small head cabbage, shredded
- 3 carrots, sliced
- 3 celery stalks, diced
- 2 cans (15 oz each) white beans, drained and rinsed
- 6 cups low-sodium vegetable broth
- 1 teaspoon dried thyme
- 1 teaspoon smoked paprika
- 1/2 teaspoon black pepper
- Salt to taste
- 1/4 cup fresh dill, chopped, for garnish

Instructions:

1. In a large pot, heat olive oil over medium heat. Add finely chopped onion and minced garlic. Sauté until the onion is translucent.

2. Add shredded cabbage, sliced carrots, and diced celery to the pot. Cook for 5-7 minutes, stirring occasionally.

3. Pour in low-sodium vegetable broth and add drained and rinsed white beans. Stir adequately.

4. Season the stew with dried thyme, smoked paprika, black pepper, and salt to taste. Bring the stew to a boil, then reduce the heat to low, cover, and simmer for 25-30 minutes or until the vegetables are tender.

5. Adjust the seasoning if necessary.

6. Serve the cabbage and white bean stew hot, garnished with chopped fresh dill.

7. Enjoy your heart-healthy DASH diet meal!

Nutritional Information (Per Serving):

- **Carbs:** 35g
- **Sodium:** 400mg
- **Phosphorus:** 250mg
- **Potassium:** 600mg
- **Protein:** 10g

Chicken and Barley Vegetable Soup

Prep Time: 20 minutes | **Cook Time:** 40 minutes | **Number of Servings:** 6

Ingredients:

- 1 pound boneless, skinless chicken breasts, diced
- 1 tablespoon olive oil
- 1 large onion, finely chopped
- 3 carrots, sliced
- 3 celery stalks, diced
- 3 cloves garlic, minced
- 1 cup pearl barley
- 8 cups low-sodium chicken broth
- 2 bay leaves
- 1 teaspoon dried thyme
- 1/2 teaspoon dried rosemary
- 1/2 teaspoon black pepper
- Salt to taste
- 2 cups green beans, trimmed and cut into 1-inch pieces
- 1 cup corn kernels (fresh or frozen)
- 1/4 cup fresh parsley, chopped, for garnish

Instructions:

1. In a large pot, heat olive oil over medium heat. Add finely chopped onion, sliced carrots, diced celery, and minced garlic. Sauté until vegetables are tender.

2. Add diced chicken to the pot and cook until browned.

3. Stir in pearl barley, low-sodium chicken broth, bay leaves, dried thyme, dried rosemary, black pepper, and salt to taste. Bring the soup to a boil.

4. Reduce the heat to low, cover, and simmer for 25-30 minutes or until the barley is tender.

5. Add green beans and corn to the pot. Continue to simmer for an additional 10 minutes until the vegetables are cooked.

6. Take out the bay leaves and discard.

7. Adjust the seasoning if necessary.

8. Serve the chicken and barley vegetable soup hot, garnished with chopped fresh parsley.

9. Enjoy your heart-healthy DASH diet meal!

Nutritional Information (Per Serving):

- **Carbs:** 40g
- **Sodium:** 400mg
- **Phosphorus:** 250mg
- **Potassium:** 600mg
- **Protein:** 25g

Tuscan White Bean and Kale Stew

Prep Time: 15 minutes | **Cook Time:** 30 minutes | **Number of Servings:** 4

Ingredients:

- 2 tablespoons olive oil
- 1 large onion, finely chopped
- 3 cloves garlic, minced
- 2 carrots, sliced
- 2 celery stalks, diced
- 1 can (14 oz) diced tomatoes, undrained
- 2 cans (15 oz each) cannellini beans, drained and rinsed
- 6 cups low-sodium vegetable broth
- 1 teaspoon dried thyme
- 1 teaspoon dried rosemary
- 1/2 teaspoon red pepper flakes (adjust to taste)
- Salt and black pepper to taste
- 4 cups kale, stems removed and leaves chopped
- 1/4 cup fresh basil, chopped, for garnish
- Grated Parmesan cheese for serving (optional)

Instructions:

1. In a large pot, heat olive oil over medium heat. Add finely chopped onion and minced garlic. Sauté until the onion is translucent.

2. Add sliced carrots and diced celery to the pot. Cook for 5 minutes, stirring occasionally.

3. Pour in diced tomatoes (with their juice), drained and rinsed cannellini beans, low-sodium vegetable broth, dried thyme, dried rosemary, red pepper flakes, salt, and black pepper. Stir adequately.

4. Bring the stew to a boil, then reduce the heat to low, cover, and simmer for 15-20 minutes.

5. Add chopped kale to the pot and simmer for an additional 5-7 minutes or until the kale is wilted.

6. Adjust the seasoning if necessary.

7. Serve the Tuscan white bean and kale stew hot, garnished with chopped fresh basil.

8. Optionally, top with grated Parmesan cheese when serving.

9. Enjoy your heart-healthy DASH diet meal!

Nutritional Information (Per Serving):

- **Carbs:** 35g
- **Sodium:** 400mg
- **Phosphorus:** 250mg
- **Potassium:** 700mg
- **Protein:** 10g

Mexican Chicken Tortilla Soup

Prep Time: 15 minutes | **Cook Time:** 30 minutes | **Number of Servings:** 6

Ingredients:

- 1 pound boneless, skinless chicken breasts, diced
- 1 tablespoon olive oil
- 1 large onion, finely chopped
- 3 cloves garlic, minced
- 1 bell pepper, diced
- 1 jalapeño, seeds removed and finely chopped
- 1 can (14 oz) diced tomatoes, undrained
- 1 can (4 oz) diced green chilies, undrained
- 6 cups low-sodium chicken broth
- 1 teaspoon ground cumin
- 1 teaspoon chili powder
- 1/2 teaspoon smoked paprika
- Salt and black pepper to taste
- 1 cup corn kernels (fresh or frozen)
- 1 can (15 oz) black beans, drained and rinsed
- 1/4 cup fresh cilantro, chopped, for garnish
- Baked tortilla strips for serving

Instructions:

1. In a large pot, heat olive oil over medium heat. Add finely chopped onion, minced garlic, diced bell pepper, and finely chopped jalapeño. Sauté until the vegetables are tender.

2. Add diced chicken to the pot and cook until browned.

3. Pour in diced tomatoes (with their juice), diced green chilies, low-sodium chicken broth, ground cumin, chili powder, smoked paprika, salt, and black pepper. Stir adequately.

4. Bring the soup to a boil, then reduce the heat to low, cover, and simmer for 20-25 minutes.

5. Add corn kernels and drained black beans to the pot. Cook for an additional 5-7 minutes.

6. Adjust the seasoning if necessary.

7. Serve the Mexican chicken tortilla soup hot, garnished with chopped fresh cilantro and baked tortilla strips.

8. Enjoy your heart-healthy DASH diet meal!

Nutritional Information (Per Serving):

- **Carbs:** 30g
- **Sodium:** 400mg
- **Phosphorus:** 250mg
- **Potassium:** 600mg
- **Protein:** 25g

Mediterranean Fish Stew

Prep Time: 20 minutes | **Cook Time:** 25 minutes | **Number of Servings:** 4

Ingredients:

- 1 pound white fish fillets (such as cod or tilapia), cut into chunks
- 2 tablespoons olive oil
- 1 large onion, finely chopped
- 3 cloves garlic, minced
- 1 fennel bulb, sliced
- 1 can (14 oz) diced tomatoes, undrained
- 1/2 cup Kalamata olives, pitted and sliced
- 1/4 cup capers, drained
- 1 teaspoon dried oregano
- 1 teaspoon dried thyme
- 1/2 teaspoon red pepper flakes (adjust to taste)
- Salt and black pepper to taste
- 1/2 cup dry white wine (optional)
- 2 cups low-sodium vegetable broth
- 1/4 cup fresh parsley, chopped, for garnish
- Lemon wedges for serving

Instructions:

1. In a large pot, heat olive oil over medium heat. Add finely chopped onion, minced garlic, and sliced fennel. Sauté until the vegetables are tender.

2. Add chunks of white fish to the pot and cook until they start to turn opaque.

3. Pour in diced tomatoes (with their juice), sliced Kalamata olives, drained capers, dried oregano, dried thyme, red pepper flakes, salt, and black pepper. Stir adequately.

4. If using, add dry white wine to the pot and let it simmer for 2-3 minutes.

5. Pour in low-sodium vegetable broth and bring the stew to a gentle simmer. Cook for 15-20 minutes or until the fish is fully cooked.

6. Adjust the seasoning if necessary.

7. Serve the Mediterranean fish stew hot, garnished with chopped fresh parsley.

8. Squeeze lemon wedges over the stew before serving.

9. Enjoy your heart-healthy DASH diet meal!

Nutritional Information (Per Serving):

- **Carbs:** 10g
- **Sodium:** 500mg
- **Phosphorus:** 200mg
- **Potassium:** 600mg
- **Protein:** 25g

Chapter 5: Salads

Greek Salad with Quinoa

Prep Time: 15 minutes | **Cook Time:** 15 minutes | **Number of Servings:** 4

Ingredients:

- 1 cup quinoa, rinsed
- 2 cups water
- 1 cucumber, diced
- 1 cup cherry tomatoes, halved
- 1/2 red onion, thinly sliced
- 1/2 cup Kalamata olives, pitted and sliced
- 1/2 cup feta cheese, crumbled
- 1/4 cup fresh parsley, chopped
- 1/4 cup extra-virgin olive oil
- 2 tablespoons red wine vinegar
- 1 teaspoon dried oregano
- Salt and pepper to taste

Instructions:

1. In a medium saucepan, combine quinoa and water. Bring to a boil, then reduce heat to low, cover, and simmer for 15 minutes, or until quinoa is cooked and water is absorbed. Fluff with a fork and let it cool.

2. In a large salad bowl, put together the cooled quinoa, cucumber, cherry tomatoes, red onion, Kalamata olives, feta cheese, and fresh parsley.

3. In a small bowl, whisk together olive oil, red wine vinegar, dried oregano, salt, and pepper. Pour the dressing over the salad and toss gently to combine.

4. Serve immediately or refrigerate for a few hours to let the flavors meld.

Nutritional Information (per serving):

- **Carbs:** 45g
- **Sodium:** 350mg
- **Phosphorus:** 200mg
- **Potassium:** 450mg
- **Protein:** 10g

<u>Avocado and Chickpea Salad</u>

Prep Time: 15 minutes | **Cook Time:** 0 minutes | **Number of Servings:** 4

Ingredients:

- 2 cans (15 oz each) chickpeas, drained and rinsed
- 2 ripe avocados, diced
- 1 cup cherry tomatoes, halved
- 1/2 red onion, finely chopped
- 1/4 cup fresh cilantro, chopped
- 1/4 cup extra-virgin olive oil
- 2 tablespoons lime juice
- 1 teaspoon ground cumin
- Salt and pepper to taste

Instructions:

1. In a large mixing bowl, put together the chickpeas, diced avocados, cherry tomatoes, red onion, and fresh cilantro.
2. In a small bowl, whisk together the olive oil, lime juice, ground cumin, salt, and pepper to create the dressing.
3. Pour the dressing over the chickpea mixture and toss gently until well coated.
4. Serve immediately or refrigerate for at least 30 minutes before serving to allow the flavors to meld.

Nutritional Information (per serving):

- **Carbs:** 40g
- **Sodium:** 300mg
- **Phosphorus:** 180mg
- **Potassium:** 600mg
- **Protein:** 10g

Spinach and Strawberry Salad

Prep Time: 10 minutes | **Cook Time:** 0 minutes | **Number of Servings:** 4

Ingredients:

- 8 cups fresh baby spinach
- 2 cups strawberries, hulled and sliced
- 1/2 cup red onion, thinly sliced
- 1/2 cup crumbled feta cheese
- 1/4 cup sliced almonds, toasted
- 1/4 cup extra-virgin olive oil
- 2 tablespoons balsamic vinegar
- 1 tablespoon honey
- Salt and pepper to taste

Instructions:

1. In a large salad bowl, put together the fresh baby spinach, sliced strawberries, thinly sliced red onion, crumbled feta cheese, and toasted sliced almonds.

2. In a small bowl, whisk together the extra-virgin olive oil, balsamic vinegar, honey, salt, and pepper to create the dressing.

3. Drizzle the dressing over the salad and toss gently until the ingredients are well coated.

4. Serve immediately to maintain the crispness of the spinach and strawberries.

Nutritional Information (per serving):

- **Carbs:** 20g
- **Sodium:** 250mg
- **Phosphorus:** 150mg
- **Potassium:** 550mg
- **Protein:** 6g

Cucumber and Tomato Salad with Feta

Prep Time: 10 minutes | **Cook Time:** 0 minutes | **Number of Servings:** 4

Ingredients:

- 4 medium cucumbers, peeled and diced
- 2 cups cherry tomatoes, halved
- 1/2 red onion, finely chopped
- 1/2 cup crumbled feta cheese
- 1/4 cup fresh dill, chopped
- 1/4 cup extra-virgin olive oil
- 2 tablespoons red wine vinegar
- 1 teaspoon dried oregano
- Salt and pepper to taste

Instructions:

1. In a large bowl, put together the diced cucumbers, halved cherry tomatoes, finely chopped red onion, crumbled feta cheese, and chopped fresh dill.
2. In a small bowl, whisk together the extra-virgin olive oil, red wine vinegar, dried oregano, salt, and pepper to create the dressing.
3. Pour the dressing over the cucumber and tomato mixture and toss gently until well combined.
4. Serve immediately or refrigerate for at least 30 minutes before serving to enhance the flavors.

Nutritional Information (per serving):

- **Carbs:** 15g
- **Sodium:** 300mg
- **Phosphorus:** 120mg
- **Potassium:** 500mg
- **Protein:** 5g

Tuna and White Bean Salad

Prep Time: 15 minutes | **Cook Time:** 0 minutes | **Number of Servings:** 4

Ingredients:

- 2 cans (15 oz each) white beans, drained and rinsed
- 2 cans (5 oz each) tuna in water, drained
- 1 red bell pepper, diced
- 1/2 red onion, finely chopped
- 1/4 cup fresh parsley, chopped
- 1/4 cup extra-virgin olive oil
- 2 tablespoons red wine vinegar
- 1 teaspoon Dijon mustard
- Salt and pepper to taste

Instructions:

1. In a large mixing bowl, put together the white beans, drained tuna, diced red bell pepper, finely chopped red onion, and chopped fresh parsley.
2. In a small bowl, whisk together the extra-virgin olive oil, red wine vinegar, Dijon mustard, salt, and pepper to create the dressing.
3. Pour the dressing over the bean and tuna mixture, tossing gently to ensure even coating.
4. Serve immediately or refrigerate for at least 30 minutes to allow the flavors to meld.

Nutritional Information (per serving):

- **Carbs:** 30g
- **Sodium:** 350mg
- **Phosphorus:** 250mg
- **Potassium:** 600mg
- **Protein:** 20g

Quinoa and Black Bean Salad

Prep Time: 15 minutes | **Cook Time:** 15 minutes | **Number of Servings:** 4

Ingredients:

- 1 cup quinoa, rinsed
- 2 cups water
- 1 can (15 oz) black beans, drained and rinsed
- 1 cup corn kernels (fresh or frozen)
- 1 red bell pepper, diced
- 1/2 red onion, finely chopped
- 1/4 cup fresh cilantro, chopped
- 1/4 cup extra-virgin olive oil
- 2 tablespoons lime juice
- 1 teaspoon ground cumin
- Salt and pepper to taste

Instructions:

1. In a medium saucepan, combine quinoa and water. Bring to a boil, then reduce heat to low, cover, and simmer for 15 minutes, or until quinoa is cooked and water is absorbed. Fluff with a fork and let it cool.

2. In a large salad bowl, put together the cooked quinoa, black beans, corn kernels, diced red bell pepper, finely chopped red onion, and chopped fresh cilantro.

3. In a small bowl, whisk together the extra-virgin olive oil, lime juice, ground cumin, salt, and pepper to create the dressing.

4. Pour the dressing over the quinoa and black bean mixture, tossing gently to ensure even coating.

5. Serve immediately or refrigerate for at least 30 minutes to allow the flavors to meld.

Nutritional Information (per serving):

- **Carbs:** 50g
- **Sodium:** 300mg
- **Phosphorus:** 250mg
- **Potassium:** 500mg
- **Protein:** 12g

Watermelon and Feta Salad

Prep Time: 15 minutes | **Cook Time:** 0 minutes | **Number of Servings:** 4

Ingredients:

- 4 cups watermelon, diced
- 1 cup cucumber, sliced
- 1 cup feta cheese, crumbled
- 1/4 cup fresh mint leaves, chopped
- 1/4 cup extra-virgin olive oil
- 2 tablespoons balsamic vinegar
- Salt and pepper to taste

Instructions:

1. In a large salad bowl, put together the diced watermelon, sliced cucumber, crumbled feta cheese, and chopped fresh mint leaves.

2. In a small bowl, whisk together the extra-virgin olive oil, balsamic vinegar, salt, and pepper to create the dressing.

3. Drizzle the dressing over the watermelon and feta mixture, tossing gently to ensure even coating.

4. Serve immediately or refrigerate for at least 30 minutes before serving to enhance the flavors.

Nutritional Information (per serving):

- **Carbs:** 20g
- **Sodium:** 300mg
- **Phosphorus:** 180mg
- **Potassium:** 400mg
- **Protein:** 8g

Lentil and Vegetable Salad

Prep Time: 20 minutes | **Cook Time:** 25 minutes | **Number of Servings:** 4

Ingredients:

- 1 cup dried green lentils
- 3 cups water
- 1 cup cherry tomatoes, halved
- 1 cucumber, diced
- 1 red bell pepper, diced
- 1/2 red onion, finely chopped
- 1/4 cup fresh parsley, chopped
- 1/4 cup extra-virgin olive oil
- 2 tablespoons red wine vinegar
- 1 teaspoon Dijon mustard
- Salt and pepper to taste

Instructions:

1. Rinse the dried green lentils under cold water. In a medium saucepan, put together the rinsed lentils and water. Bring to a boil, then reduce heat to low, cover, and simmer for 25 minutes or until lentils are tender. Drain any excess water and let them cool.

2. In a large salad bowl, put together the cooked lentils, halved cherry tomatoes, diced cucumber, diced red bell pepper, finely chopped red onion, and chopped fresh parsley.

3. In a small bowl, whisk together the extra-virgin olive oil, red wine vinegar, Dijon mustard, salt, and pepper to create the dressing.

4. Pour the dressing over the lentil and vegetable mixture, tossing gently to ensure even coating.

5. Serve immediately or refrigerate for at least 30 minutes before serving to allow the flavors to meld.

Nutritional Information (per serving):

- **Carbs:** 40g
- **Sodium:** 300mg
- **Phosphorus:** 250mg
- **Potassium:** 600mg
- **Protein:** 15g

<u>Citrus and Arugula Salad</u>

Prep Time: 15 minutes | **Cook Time:** 0 minutes | **Number of Servings:** 4

Ingredients:

- 6 cups arugula, washed and dried
- 2 oranges, peeled and segmented
- 1 grapefruit, peeled and segmented
- 1 avocado, sliced
- 1/4 cup red onion, thinly sliced
- 1/4 cup almonds, toasted
- 1/4 cup extra-virgin olive oil
- 2 tablespoons balsamic vinegar
- 1 teaspoon honey
- Salt and pepper to taste

Instructions:

1. In a large salad bowl, put together the washed and dried arugula, peeled and segmented oranges, peeled and segmented grapefruit, sliced avocado, thinly sliced red onion, and toasted almonds.

2. In a small bowl, whisk together the extra-virgin olive oil, balsamic vinegar, honey, salt, and pepper to create the dressing.

3. Drizzle the dressing over the arugula and citrus mixture, tossing gently to ensure even coating.

4. Serve immediately to maintain the freshness of the arugula and citrus.

Nutritional Information (per serving):

- **Carbs:** 25g
- **Sodium:** 150mg
- **Phosphorus:** 150mg
- **Potassium:** 600mg
- **Protein:** 5g

Roasted Vegetable and Farro Salad

Prep Time: 20 minutes | **Cook Time:** 30 minutes | **Number of Servings:** 4

Ingredients:

- 1 cup farro
- 2 cups water
- 2 cups mixed vegetables (zucchini, bell peppers, cherry tomatoes), diced
- 1 red onion, sliced
- 1 tablespoon olive oil
- Salt and pepper to taste
- 1/4 cup fresh basil, chopped
- 1/4 cup feta cheese, crumbled
- 2 tablespoons balsamic vinegar

Instructions:

1. In a medium saucepan, combine farro and water. Bring to a boil, then reduce heat to low, cover, and simmer for 30 minutes or until farro is tender. Drain any excess water and let it cool.

2. Preheat the oven to 400°F (200°C). In a baking sheet, toss the diced mixed vegetables and sliced red onion with olive oil, salt, and pepper. Roast in the preheated oven for 20-25 minutes or until the vegetables are tender and slightly caramelized.

3. In a large salad bowl, put together the cooked farro, roasted mixed vegetables and red onion, chopped fresh basil, and crumbled feta cheese.

4. Drizzle balsamic vinegar over the salad and toss gently to combine.

5. Serve immediately or refrigerate for at least 30 minutes before serving to allow the flavors to meld.

Nutritional Information (per serving):

- **Carbs:** 45g
- **Sodium:** 250mg
- **Phosphorus:** 200mg
- **Potassium:** 400mg
- **Protein:** 8g

Kale and Cranberry Salad

Prep Time: 15 minutes | **Cook Time:** 0 minutes | **Number of Servings:** 4

Ingredients:

- 1 bunch kale, stems removed, leaves chopped
- 1/2 cup dried cranberries
- 1/4 cup sunflower seeds
- 1/4 cup feta cheese, crumbled
- 1/4 cup red onion, thinly sliced
- 1/4 cup extra-virgin olive oil
- 2 tablespoons apple cider vinegar
- 1 teaspoon Dijon mustard
- Salt and pepper to taste

Instructions:

1. In a large salad bowl, put together the chopped kale, dried cranberries, sunflower seeds, crumbled feta cheese, and thinly sliced red onion.

2. In a small bowl, whisk together the extra-virgin olive oil, apple cider vinegar, Dijon mustard, salt, and pepper to create the dressing.

3. Pour the dressing over the kale and cranberry mixture, tossing gently to ensure even coating.

4. Allow the salad to sit for at least 10 minutes to allow the kale to soften slightly.

5. Serve immediately or refrigerate for up to 30 minutes before serving.

Nutritional Information (per serving):

- **Carbs:** 20g
- **Sodium:** 200mg
- **Phosphorus:** 120mg
- **Potassium:** 400mg
- **Protein:** 5g

Caprese Salad with Whole Wheat Croutons

Prep Time: 15 minutes | **Cook Time:** 10 minutes | **Number of Servings:** 4

Ingredients:

- 4 slices whole wheat bread, cut into cubes
- 2 tablespoons olive oil
- 2 large tomatoes, sliced
- 1 ball fresh mozzarella cheese, sliced
- 1/4 cup fresh basil leaves
- 2 tablespoons balsamic glaze
- Salt and pepper to taste

Instructions:

1. Preheat the oven to 375°F (190°C).
2. In a large mixing bowl, toss the whole wheat bread cubes with olive oil until evenly coated. Spread the cubes on a baking sheet and bake for 8-10 minutes or until the croutons are golden and crispy. Allow them to cool.
3. On a serving platter, arrange the sliced tomatoes, fresh mozzarella cheese, and whole wheat croutons.
4. Tuck fresh basil leaves among the tomatoes and mozzarella.
5. Drizzle balsamic glaze over the salad, and season with salt and pepper to taste.
6. Serve immediately, allowing the croutons to maintain their crispiness.

Nutritional Information (per serving):

- **Carbs:** 30g
- **Sodium:** 300mg
- **Phosphorus:** 200mg
- **Potassium:** 400mg
- **Protein:** 12g

Asian Edamame and Noodle Salad

Prep Time: 20 minutes | **Cook Time:** 8 minutes | **Number of Servings:** 4

Ingredients:

- 8 oz whole wheat spaghetti
- 1 cup edamame, shelled
- 1 red bell pepper, julienned
- 1 carrot, julienned
- 1 cucumber, julienned
- 1/4 cup green onions, sliced
- 1/4 cup cilantro leaves, chopped
- 1/4 cup unsalted peanuts, crushed (optional)

For the Dressing:

- 3 tablespoons low-sodium soy sauce
- 2 tablespoons rice vinegar
- 1 tablespoon sesame oil
- 1 tablespoon honey
- 1 teaspoon fresh ginger, grated
- 1 clove garlic, minced

Instructions:

1. Cook the whole wheat spaghetti according to package instructions. Drain and rinse under cold water to cool.

2. In a pot of boiling water, cook the shelled edamame for 3-5 minutes. Drain and rinse with cold water.

3. In a large salad bowl, put together the cooked whole wheat spaghetti, edamame, julienned red bell pepper, julienned carrot, julienned cucumber, sliced green onions, and chopped cilantro leaves.

4. In a small bowl, whisk together the low-sodium soy sauce, rice vinegar, sesame oil, honey, grated fresh ginger, and minced garlic to create the dressing.

5. Pour the dressing over the noodle and vegetable mixture, tossing gently to ensure even coating.

6. Garnish the salad with crushed unsalted peanuts if desired.

7. Serve immediately or refrigerate for at least 30 minutes before serving to allow the flavors to meld.

Nutritional Information (per serving):

- **Carbs:** 45g
- **Sodium:** 400mg
- **Phosphorus:** 200mg
- **Potassium:** 550mg
- **Protein:** 15g

Pomegranate and Walnut Spinach Salad

Prep Time: 15 minutes | **Cook Time:** 0 minutes | **Number of Servings:** 4

Ingredients:

- 8 cups fresh baby spinach
- 1 cup pomegranate seeds
- 1/2 cup walnuts, chopped
- 1/4 cup red onion, thinly sliced
- 1/4 cup feta cheese, crumbled
- 1/4 cup extra-virgin olive oil
- 2 tablespoons balsamic vinegar
- 1 teaspoon honey
- Salt and pepper to taste

Instructions:

1. In a large salad bowl, put together the fresh baby spinach, pomegranate seeds, chopped walnuts, thinly sliced red onion, and crumbled feta cheese.

2. In a small bowl, whisk together the extra-virgin olive oil, balsamic vinegar, honey, salt, and pepper to create the dressing.

3. Drizzle the dressing over the spinach and pomegranate mixture, tossing gently to ensure even coating.

4. Serve immediately to maintain the crispness of the spinach.

Nutritional Information (per serving):

- **Carbs:** 20g
- **Sodium:** 250mg
- **Phosphorus:** 150mg
- **Potassium:** 600mg
- **Protein:** 6g

Shrimp and Avocado Salad

Prep Time: 15 minutes | **Cook Time:** 5 minutes | **Number of Servings:** 4

Ingredients:

- 1 lb large shrimp, peeled and deveined
- 2 avocados, diced
- 1 cup cherry tomatoes, halved
- 1/4 cup red onion, finely chopped
- 1/4 cup fresh cilantro, chopped
- 1/4 cup extra-virgin olive oil
- 2 tablespoons lime juice
- 1 teaspoon cumin
- Salt and pepper to taste
- Mixed salad greens for serving

Instructions:

1. In a skillet over medium heat, cook the peeled and deveined shrimp for 3-5 minutes until opaque and cooked through. Set aside to cool.

2. In a large mixing bowl, put together the diced avocados, halved cherry tomatoes, finely chopped red onion, and chopped fresh cilantro.

3. Add the cooked shrimp to the bowl with the avocado mixture.

4. In a small bowl, whisk together the extra-virgin olive oil, lime juice, cumin, salt, and pepper to create the dressing.

5. Pour the dressing over the shrimp and avocado mixture, tossing gently to ensure even coating.

6. Serve the shrimp and avocado mixture over a bed of mixed salad greens.

Nutritional Information (per serving):

- **Carbs:** 15g
- **Sodium:** 300mg
- **Phosphorus:** 250mg
- **Potassium:** 600mg
- **Protein:** 25g

Caesar Salad with Grilled Chicken

Prep Time: 20 minutes | **Cook Time:** 15 minutes | **Number of Servings:** 4

Ingredients:

- 2 boneless, skinless chicken breasts
- 1 tablespoon olive oil
- Salt and black pepper to taste
- 2 hearts of romaine lettuce, chopped
- 1 cup cherry tomatoes, halved
- 1/2 cup croutons
- 1/2 cup grated Parmesan cheese

For the Caesar Dressing:

- 1/2 cup plain Greek yogurt
- 2 tablespoons olive oil
- 2 tablespoons lemon juice
- 1 tablespoon Dijon mustard
- 2 cloves garlic, minced
- Salt and black pepper to taste

Instructions:

1. Preheat a grill or grill pan over medium-high heat.

2. Rub the chicken breasts with olive oil and season with salt and black pepper. Grill for about 6-8 minutes per side or until fully cooked. Allow the chicken to rest before slicing it into strips.

3. In a large salad bowl, put together the chopped romaine lettuce, halved cherry tomatoes, croutons, and grated Parmesan cheese.

4. In a small bowl, whisk together the Greek yogurt, olive oil, lemon juice, Dijon mustard, minced garlic, salt, and black pepper to create the Caesar dressing.

5. Pour the Caesar dressing over the salad and toss gently to coat the ingredients.

6. Top the salad with grilled chicken strips.

7. Serve immediately.

Nutritional Information (per serving):

- **Carbs:** 15g
- **Sodium:** 400mg
- **Phosphorus:** 200mg
- **Potassium:** 500mg
- **Protein:** 25g

Mango and Quinoa Salad

Prep Time: 15 minutes | **Cook Time:** 15 minutes | **Number of Servings:** 4

Ingredients:

- 1 cup quinoa, rinsed
- 2 cups water
- 2 ripe mangos, diced
- 1 red bell pepper, diced
- 1/2 red onion, finely chopped
- 1/4 cup fresh cilantro, chopped
- 1/4 cup lime juice
- 2 tablespoons extra-virgin olive oil
- Salt and black pepper to taste
- Mixed salad greens for serving

Instructions:

1. In a medium saucepan, combine quinoa and water. Bring to a boil, then reduce heat to low, cover, and simmer for 15 minutes or until quinoa is cooked and water is absorbed. Fluff with a fork and let it cool.

2. In a large salad bowl, put together the cooked quinoa, diced ripe mangos, diced red bell pepper, finely chopped red onion, and chopped fresh cilantro.

3. In a small bowl, whisk together the lime juice, extra-virgin olive oil, salt, and black pepper to create the dressing.

4. Pour the dressing over the quinoa and mango mixture, tossing gently to ensure even coating.

5. Serve the salad over a bed of mixed salad greens.

Nutritional Information (per serving):

- **Carbs:** 45g
- **Sodium:** 200mg
- **Phosphorus:** 250mg
- **Potassium:** 600mg
- **Protein:** 8g

Broccoli and Almond Salad

Prep Time: 15 minutes | **Cook Time:** 5 minutes | **Number of Servings:** 4

Ingredients:

- 4 cups broccoli florets, blanched
- 1/2 cup almonds, sliced and toasted
- 1/4 cup red onion, finely chopped
- 1/4 cup dried cranberries
- 1/4 cup feta cheese, crumbled
- 1/4 cup plain Greek yogurt
- 2 tablespoons mayonnaise
- 1 tablespoon apple cider vinegar
- 1 tablespoon honey
- Salt and black pepper to taste

Instructions:

1. In a large mixing bowl, put together the blanched broccoli florets, sliced and toasted almonds, finely chopped red onion, dried cranberries, and crumbled feta cheese.

2. In a small bowl, whisk together the plain Greek yogurt, mayonnaise, apple cider vinegar, honey, salt, and black pepper to create the dressing.

3. Pour the dressing over the broccoli and almond mixture, tossing gently to ensure even coating.

4. Allow the salad to chill in the refrigerator for at least 30 minutes before serving.

5. Serve the broccoli and almond salad as a refreshing side dish.

Nutritional Information (per serving):

- **Carbs:** 20g
- **Sodium:** 300mg
- **Phosphorus:** 150mg
- **Potassium:** 500mg
- **Protein:** 8g

Chapter 6: Main Dishes

Grilled Lemon Herb Chicken

Prep Time: 15 minutes | Cook Time: 20 minutes | Servings: 4

Ingredients:

- 4 boneless, skinless chicken breasts
- 2 lemons, juiced and zested
- 3 cloves garlic, minced
- 2 tablespoons fresh rosemary, chopped
- 2 tablespoons fresh thyme, chopped
- 2 tablespoons olive oil
- Salt and pepper to taste

Instructions:

1. In a small bowl, put together the lemon juice, lemon zest, minced garlic, chopped rosemary, chopped thyme, olive oil, salt, and pepper. Mix adequately to create the marinade.

2. Place the chicken breasts in a shallow dish and pour half of the marinade over them. Ensure each breast is well coated. Cover the dish and refrigerate for at least 1 hour to let the flavors infuse.

3. Preheat the grill to medium-high heat.

4. Take out the chicken from the refrigerator and let it come to room temperature for about 10 minutes.

5. Grill the chicken for approximately 8-10 minutes per side or until the internal temperature reaches 165°F (74°C). Baste the chicken with the remaining marinade during grilling.

6. Once cooked, take out the chicken from the grill and let it rest for a few minutes before serving.

Nutritional Information (Per Serving):

- **Carbs:** 3g
- **Sodium:** 450mg
- **Phosphorus:** 230mg
- **Potassium:** 380mg
- **Protein:** 25g

Baked Salmon with Dill Sauce

Prep Time: 15 minutes | Cook Time: 20 minutes | Servings: 4

Ingredients:

- 4 salmon fillets
- 1 lemon, sliced
- 2 tablespoons fresh dill, chopped
- 2 cloves garlic, minced
- 1/4 cup low-sodium vegetable broth
- 1/4 cup plain Greek yogurt
- Salt and pepper to taste

Instructions:

1. Preheat the oven to 375°F (190°C). Line a baking sheet with parchment paper.

2. Place the salmon fillets on the prepared baking sheet. Season each fillet with salt and pepper to taste. Top each fillet with lemon slices.

3. In a small bowl, mix together chopped dill, minced garlic, vegetable broth, and Greek yogurt to create the dill sauce.

4. Spoon the dill sauce evenly over each salmon fillet, ensuring they are well-covered.

5. Bake in the preheated oven for about 15-20 minutes or until the salmon is cooked through and flakes easily with a fork.

6. While the salmon is baking, prepare a side dish of steamed vegetables or a green salad to complement the meal.

Nutritional Information (Per Serving):

- **Carbs:** 3g
- **Sodium:** 180mg
- **Phosphorus:** 320mg
- **Potassium:** 450mg
- **Protein:** 30g

Turkey and Quinoa Stuffed Peppers

Prep Time: 20 minutes | Cook Time: 40 minutes | Servings: 6

Ingredients:

- 1 cup quinoa, rinsed
- 6 bell peppers, halved and seeds removed
- 1 lb ground turkey
- 1 onion, finely chopped
- 2 cloves garlic, minced
- 1 can (15 oz) low-sodium black beans, drained and rinsed
- 1 can (14 oz) diced tomatoes, drained
- 1 teaspoon ground cumin
- 1 teaspoon chili powder
- 1/2 teaspoon paprika
- Salt and pepper to taste
- 1 cup low-fat shredded cheddar cheese
- Fresh cilantro for garnish (optional)

Instructions:

1. Preheat the oven to 375°F (190°C).
2. In a medium saucepan, cook the quinoa according to package instructions. Set aside.
3. Place the halved bell peppers in a baking dish, cut side up.
4. In a large skillet, cook the ground turkey over medium heat until browned. Add finely chopped onion and minced garlic, cooking until the onion is soft.
5. Stir in the drained black beans, drained diced tomatoes, ground cumin, chili powder, paprika, salt, and pepper. Allow the mixture to simmer for 5-7 minutes.
6. Add the cooked quinoa to the turkey mixture, combining well.
7. Spoon the turkey and quinoa mixture evenly into each bell pepper half.
8. Top each stuffed pepper with shredded cheddar cheese.
9. Cover the baking dish with aluminum foil and bake in the preheated oven for 25-30 minutes or until the peppers are tender.
10. If desired, garnish with fresh cilantro before serving.

Nutritional Information (Per Serving):

- **Carbs:** 35g
- **Sodium:** 320mg
- **Phosphorus:** 380mg
- **Potassium:** 650mg
- **Protein:** 25g

Eggplant and Lentil Moussaka

Prep Time: 30 minutes | Cook Time: 1 hour | Servings: 8

Ingredients:

- 2 large eggplants, sliced into 1/2-inch rounds
- 1 cup dried green lentils, rinsed
- 1 can (14 oz) diced tomatoes
- 1 onion, finely chopped
- 3 cloves garlic, minced
- 2 teaspoons dried oregano
- 2 teaspoons dried thyme
- 1 teaspoon ground cinnamon
- 1/2 teaspoon ground nutmeg
- 2 tablespoons tomato paste
- 2 tablespoons olive oil
- 1 cup low-fat milk
- 2 tablespoons all-purpose flour
- Salt and pepper to taste
- 1/2 cup grated Parmesan cheese (optional)

Instructions:

1. Preheat the oven to 400°F (200°C). Place eggplant slices on a baking sheet, brush with olive oil, and bake for 20-25 minutes or until tender. Set aside.

2. In a medium saucepan, put together the rinsed lentils with enough water to cover them. Bring to a boil, then reduce heat and simmer for 20-25 minutes, or until lentils are tender. Drain any excess water.

3. In a separate pan, sauté finely chopped onion and minced garlic until softened. Add diced tomatoes, dried oregano, dried thyme, ground cinnamon, ground nutmeg, and tomato paste. Cook for an additional 5-7 minutes.

4. Combine the cooked lentils with the tomato mixture.

5. In a small saucepan, whisk together low-fat milk and all-purpose flour to create a béchamel sauce. Cook over medium heat until thickened. Season with salt and pepper.

6. In a baking dish, layer half of the eggplant slices, followed by the lentil and tomato mixture. Repeat the layers, finishing with a layer of eggplant on top.

7. Pour the béchamel sauce over the top layer of eggplant, spreading it evenly.

8. If desired, sprinkle with grated Parmesan cheese.

9. Bake in the preheated oven for 30-40 minutes, or until the top is golden brown.

Nutritional Information (Per Serving):

- **Carbs:** 35g
- **Sodium:** 320mg
- **Phosphorus:** 300mg
- **Potassium:** 580mg
- **Protein:** 15g

Shrimp and Vegetable Stir-Fry

Prep Time: 20 minutes | Cook Time: 10 minutes | Servings: 4

Ingredients:

- 1 lb large shrimp, peeled and deveined
- 2 cups broccoli florets
- 1 red bell pepper, thinly sliced
- 1 yellow bell pepper, thinly sliced
- 1 carrot, julienned
- 1 cup snap peas, ends trimmed
- 3 cloves garlic, minced
- 1 tablespoon fresh ginger, grated
- 1/4 cup low-sodium soy sauce
- 2 tablespoons rice vinegar
- 1 tablespoon honey
- 1 tablespoon cornstarch
- 2 tablespoons canola oil
- Sesame seeds for garnish (optional)
- Green onions, sliced, for garnish (optional)

Instructions:

1. In a small bowl, whisk together low-sodium soy sauce, rice vinegar, honey, and cornstarch to create the sauce. Set aside.

2. Heat canola oil in a wok or large skillet over medium-high heat.

3. Add minced garlic and grated ginger to the hot oil, stirring constantly for about 30 seconds or until fragrant.

4. Add peeled and deveined shrimp to the wok, cooking for 2-3 minutes or until they start to turn pink.

5. Add broccoli florets, thinly sliced red and yellow bell peppers, julienned carrot, and snap peas to the wok. Stir-fry for an additional 3-4 minutes or until the vegetables are crisp-tender.

6. Pour the prepared sauce over the shrimp and vegetables. Stir to coat evenly and cook for an additional 1-2 minutes until the sauce thickens.

7. If desired, garnish the stir-fry with sesame seeds and sliced green onions.

Nutritional Information (Per Serving):

- **Carbs:** 20g
- **Sodium:** 480mg
- **Phosphorus:** 220mg
- **Potassium:** 400mg
- **Protein:** 25g

<u>Chickpea and Vegetable Curry</u>

Prep Time: 15 minutes | Cook Time: 25 minutes | Servings: 6

Ingredients:

- 2 cans (15 oz each) chickpeas, drained and rinsed
- 1 large sweet potato, peeled and diced
- 1 cup green beans, trimmed and cut into bite-sized pieces
- 1 red bell pepper, diced
- 1 onion, finely chopped
- 3 cloves garlic, minced
- 1 tablespoon fresh ginger, grated
- 1 can (14 oz) diced tomatoes
-

- 1 can (14 oz) light coconut milk
- 2 tablespoons curry powder
- 1 teaspoon ground turmeric
- 1 teaspoon ground cumin
- 1/2 teaspoon cayenne pepper (optional)
- Salt and pepper to taste
- 2 tablespoons olive oil
- Fresh cilantro for garnish (optional)
- Brown rice or quinoa for serving

Instructions:

1. In a large pot, heat olive oil over medium heat. Add finely chopped onion, minced garlic, and grated ginger. Sauté until the onion is translucent and fragrant.

2. Add diced sweet potato, diced red bell pepper, and trimmed green beans to the pot. Cook for 5-7 minutes, stirring occasionally.

3. Sprinkle curry powder, ground turmeric, ground cumin, and cayenne pepper (if using) over the vegetables. Stir to coat the vegetables in the spices.

4. Pour in diced tomatoes (with their juice) and light coconut milk. Bring the mixture to a simmer.

5. Add drained and rinsed chickpeas to the pot, stirring to combine.

6. Season with salt and pepper to taste. Cover the pot and let it simmer for 15-20 minutes or until the sweet potatoes are tender.

7. If the curry is too thick, you can add a little water to reach your desired consistency.

8. Serve the chickpea and vegetable curry over brown rice or quinoa.

9. Garnish with fresh cilantro if desired.

Nutritional Information (Per Serving):

- **Carbs:** 40g
- **Sodium:** 380mg
- **Phosphorus:** 280mg

- **Potassium:** 600mg
- **Protein:** 15g

Lemon Garlic Herb Tilapia

Prep Time: 10 minutes | Cook Time: 15 minutes | Servings: 4

Ingredients:

- 4 tilapia fillets
- 2 lemons, juiced
- 4 cloves garlic, minced
- 2 tablespoons fresh parsley, chopped
- 1 tablespoon fresh thyme, chopped
- 1 tablespoon fresh rosemary, chopped
- 3 tablespoons olive oil
- Salt and pepper to taste
- Lemon slices for garnish (optional)

Instructions:

1. Preheat the oven to 375°F (190°C). Line a baking sheet with parchment paper.

2. Place the tilapia fillets on the prepared baking sheet.

3. In a small bowl, put together the freshly squeezed lemon juice, minced garlic, chopped parsley, chopped thyme, chopped rosemary, olive oil, salt, and pepper. Mix adequately to create the herb marinade.

4. Spoon the herb marinade over each tilapia fillet, ensuring they are well coated. Allow the fillets to marinate for 5-10 minutes.

5. Bake the tilapia in the preheated oven for 12-15 minutes or until the fish flakes easily with a fork.

6. While baking, baste the fillets with the marinade halfway through the cooking time.

7. Once done, take out the tilapia from the oven and let it rest for a few minutes before serving.

8. Garnish with lemon slices if desired.

Nutritional Information (Per Serving):

- **Carbs:** 3g
- **Sodium:** 150mg
- **Phosphorus:** 200mg
- **Potassium:** 320mg
- **Protein:** 25g

Quinoa and Black Bean Enchiladas

Prep Time: 20 minutes | Cook Time: 25 minutes | Servings: 6

Ingredients:

- 1 cup quinoa, rinsed
- 2 cups black beans, cooked and mashed
- 1 cup corn kernels (fresh or frozen)
- 1 red bell pepper, diced
- 1 onion, finely chopped
- 2 cloves garlic, minced
- 1 can (14 oz) diced tomatoes, drained
- 1 teaspoon ground cumin
- 1 teaspoon chili powder
- 1/2 teaspoon smoked paprika
- Salt and pepper to taste
- 12 whole wheat tortillas
- 2 cups enchilada sauce (store-bought or homemade)
- 1 cup shredded low-fat cheddar cheese
- Fresh cilantro for garnish (optional)
- Greek yogurt or low-fat sour cream for serving (optional)

Instructions:

1. Preheat the oven to 375°F (190°C). Grease a baking dish with olive oil or cooking spray.
2. In a medium saucepan, cook the quinoa according to package instructions. Set aside.
3. In a large mixing bowl, put together the cooked and mashed black beans, corn kernels, diced red bell pepper, finely chopped onion, minced garlic, drained diced tomatoes, ground cumin, chili powder, smoked paprika, salt, and pepper. Mix adequately.
4. Stir in the cooked quinoa into the black bean mixture.
5. Warm the whole wheat tortillas slightly to make them pliable.
6. Spoon a generous portion of the quinoa and black bean mixture onto each tortilla. Roll them up and place them seam side down in the prepared baking dish.
7. Pour the enchilada sauce over the rolled tortillas, ensuring they are well covered.
8. Sprinkle shredded low-fat cheddar cheese over the top.
9. Bake in the preheated oven for 20-25 minutes or until the cheese is melted and bubbly.
10. Garnish with fresh cilantro if desired and serve with a dollop of Greek yogurt or low-fat sour cream.

Nutritional Information (Per Serving):

- **Carbs:** 50g
- **Sodium:** 650mg
- **Phosphorus:** 320mg
- **Potassium:** 600mg
- **Protein:** 15g

Baked Chicken with Mediterranean Salsa

Prep Time: 15 minutes | Cook Time: 25 minutes | Servings: 4

Ingredients:

- 4 boneless, skinless chicken breasts
- 1 teaspoon dried oregano
- 1 teaspoon dried thyme
- 1 teaspoon garlic powder
- Salt and pepper to taste
- 2 tablespoons olive oil

Mediterranean Salsa:

- 1 cup cherry tomatoes, halved
- 1 cucumber, diced
- 1/2 red onion, finely chopped
- 1/4 cup Kalamata olives, sliced
- 2 tablespoons fresh parsley, chopped
- 2 tablespoons feta cheese, crumbled
- 2 tablespoons extra-virgin olive oil
- 1 tablespoon red wine vinegar
- Salt and pepper to taste

Instructions:

1. Preheat the oven to 400°F (200°C). Line a baking sheet with parchment paper.

2. In a small bowl, mix dried oregano, dried thyme, garlic powder, salt, and pepper. Rub the chicken breasts with the spice mixture.

3. Heat olive oil in a skillet over medium-high heat. Sear the chicken breasts for 2-3 minutes on each side until browned.

4. Transfer the seared chicken breasts to the prepared baking sheet and bake in the preheated oven for 20-25 minutes or until the internal temperature reaches 165°F (74°C).

5. While the chicken is baking, prepare the Mediterranean salsa.

6. In a bowl, combine halved cherry tomatoes, diced cucumber, finely chopped red onion, sliced Kalamata olives, chopped fresh parsley, crumbled feta cheese, extra-virgin olive oil, red wine vinegar, salt, and pepper. Mix adequately.

7. Once the chicken is done baking, serve each breast topped with a generous spoonful of Mediterranean salsa.

Nutritional Information (Per Serving):

- **Carbs:** 10g
- **Sodium:** 350mg
- **Phosphorus:** 250mg
- **Potassium:** 450mg
- **Protein:** 30g

Spinach and Mushroom Stuffed Chicken
Prep Time: 20 minutes | Cook Time: 30 minutes | Servings: 4

Ingredients:

- 4 boneless, skinless chicken breasts
- 2 cups fresh spinach, chopped
- 1 cup mushrooms, finely diced
- 1/2 cup low-fat feta cheese, crumbled
- 2 cloves garlic, minced
- 1 teaspoon dried oregano
- 1 teaspoon dried thyme
- Salt and pepper to taste
- 2 tablespoons olive oil

Instructions:

1. Preheat the oven to 375°F (190°C). Line a baking sheet with parchment paper.

2. In a skillet, heat olive oil over medium heat. Add minced garlic and sauté until fragrant.

3. Add finely diced mushrooms to the skillet and cook until they release their moisture and become tender.

4. Stir in chopped fresh spinach and cook until wilted. Remove from heat.

5. In a bowl, put together the cooked spinach and mushrooms with crumbled low-fat feta cheese, dried oregano, dried thyme, salt, and pepper. Mix adequately to create the stuffing.

6. Lay the chicken breasts on a clean surface. Cut a pocket into each chicken breast, being careful not to cut through the other side.

7. Stuff each chicken breast with the spinach and mushroom mixture.

8. Season the outside of the chicken breasts with a little salt and pepper.

9. Place the stuffed chicken breasts on the prepared baking sheet.

10. Bake in the preheated oven for 25-30 minutes or until the chicken is cooked through.

Nutritional Information (Per Serving):

- **Carbs:** 5g
- **Sodium:** 350mg
- **Phosphorus:** 250mg
- **Potassium:** 500mg
- **Protein:** 30g

Spaghetti Squash with Turkey Bolognese

Prep Time: 20 minutes | Cook Time: 45 minutes | Servings: 4

Ingredients:

- 1 medium-sized spaghetti squash
- 1 lb ground turkey
- 1 onion, finely chopped
- 2 cloves garlic, minced
- 1 carrot, grated
- 1 celery stalk, finely chopped
- 1 can (14 oz) crushed tomatoes
- 1 tablespoon tomato paste
- 1 teaspoon dried oregano
- 1 teaspoon dried basil
- 1/2 teaspoon dried thyme
- Salt and pepper to taste
- 2 tablespoons olive oil
- Fresh parsley for garnish (optional)
- Grated Parmesan cheese for serving (optional)

Instructions:

1. Preheat the oven to 400°F (200°C). Cut the spaghetti squash in half lengthwise and scoop out the seeds.

2. Place the squash halves, cut side down, on a baking sheet. Bake in the preheated oven for 35-40 minutes or until the squash is tender.

3. While the squash is baking, heat olive oil in a large skillet over medium heat. Add finely chopped onion, minced garlic, grated carrot, and finely chopped celery. Sauté until the vegetables are softened.

4. Add ground turkey to the skillet, breaking it apart with a spoon, and cook until browned.

5. Stir in crushed tomatoes, tomato paste, dried oregano, dried basil, dried thyme, salt, and pepper. Simmer for 15-20 minutes, allowing the flavors to meld.

6. Once the spaghetti squash is done baking, use a fork to scrape the flesh into "spaghetti" strands.

7. Serve the turkey bolognese over the spaghetti squash.

8. Garnish with fresh parsley and grated Parmesan cheese if desired.

Nutritional Information (Per Serving):

- **Carbs:** 20g
- **Sodium:** 480mg
- **Phosphorus:** 300mg
- **Potassium:** 600mg
- **Protein:** 25g

Tofu and Vegetable Skewers

Prep Time: 30 minutes | Cook Time: 15 minutes | Servings: 4

Ingredients:

- 1 block (14 oz) extra-firm tofu, pressed and cubed
- 1 zucchini, sliced into rounds
- 1 red bell pepper, cut into chunks
- 1 yellow bell pepper, cut into chunks
- 1 red onion, cut into wedges
- 1 cup cherry tomatoes
- 2 tablespoons olive oil
- 2 tablespoons soy sauce (low-sodium)
- 1 tablespoon balsamic vinegar
- 1 teaspoon dried oregano
- 1 teaspoon dried thyme
- 1/2 teaspoon garlic powder
- Salt and pepper to taste
- Wooden skewers, soaked in water

Instructions:

1. Press the tofu to remove excess water by wrapping it in a clean kitchen towel and placing a heavy object on top. Cut the pressed tofu into cubes.

2. In a bowl, whisk together olive oil, low-sodium soy sauce, balsamic vinegar, dried oregano, dried thyme, garlic powder, salt, and pepper to create the marinade.

3. Place the cubed tofu in the marinade, ensuring each piece is coated. Allow it to marinate for at least 15 minutes.

4. Preheat the grill or grill pan over medium-high heat.

5. Thread the marinated tofu cubes, zucchini rounds, red and yellow bell pepper chunks, red onion wedges, and cherry tomatoes onto the soaked wooden skewers.

6. Grill the skewers for 10-15 minutes, turning occasionally, until the tofu is golden brown and the vegetables are tender.

7. While grilling, brush the skewers with any remaining marinade to enhance flavor.

8. Once done, take out the skewers from the grill.

9. Serve the tofu and vegetable skewers on a bed of quinoa or brown rice if desired.

Nutritional Information (Per Serving):

- **Carbs:** 20g
- **Sodium:** 350mg
- **Phosphorus:** 300mg
- **Potassium:** 550mg
- **Protein:** 15g

Zucchini Noodles with Pesto Shrimp

Prep Time: 20 minutes | Cook Time: 10 minutes | Servings: 4

Ingredients:

- 1 lb large shrimp, peeled and deveined
- 4 medium-sized zucchini
- 1 cup cherry tomatoes, halved
- 1/2 cup grated Parmesan cheese
- 2 tablespoons pine nuts, toasted
- Fresh basil leaves for garnish

Pesto Sauce:

- 2 cups fresh basil leaves
- 1/2 cup grated Parmesan cheese
- 1/2 cup extra-virgin olive oil
- 1/4 cup pine nuts, toasted
- 2 cloves garlic, minced
- Salt and pepper to taste

Instructions:

1. In a food processor, combine fresh basil leaves, grated Parmesan cheese, toasted pine nuts, minced garlic, salt, and pepper. With the processor running, slowly pour in the extra-virgin olive oil until the pesto sauce is well blended. Set aside.

2. Using a spiralizer, create zucchini noodles from the medium-sized zucchini. If you don't have a spiralizer, you can use a julienne peeler or buy pre-spiralized zucchini noodles.

3. Heat a large skillet over medium heat. Add the peeled and deveined shrimp to the skillet, cooking for 2-3 minutes on each side until they turn pink. Remove from the skillet and set aside.

4. In the same skillet, add the zucchini noodles and cherry tomatoes. Sauté for 2-3 minutes until the noodles are just tender.

5. Add the cooked shrimp back to the skillet, along with the prepared pesto sauce. Toss everything together until well combined and heated through.

6. Take out the skillet from the heat and sprinkle grated Parmesan cheese over the zucchini noodles and shrimp.

7. Garnish with toasted pine nuts and fresh basil leaves.

8. Serve immediately.

Nutritional Information (Per Serving):

- **Carbs:** 15g
- **Sodium:** 450mg
- **Phosphorus:** 200mg
- **Potassium:** 550mg
- **Protein:** 25g

Cabbage and Turkey Sauté

Prep Time: 15 minutes | Cook Time: 20 minutes | Servings: 4

Ingredients:

- 1 lb ground turkey
- 1 small head cabbage, shredded
- 1 onion, thinly sliced
- 2 carrots, julienned
- 3 cloves garlic, minced
- 1 teaspoon dried thyme
- 1 teaspoon paprika
- 1/2 teaspoon caraway seeds
- Salt and pepper to taste
- 2 tablespoons olive oil
- Fresh parsley for garnish (optional)

Instructions:

1. In a large skillet, heat olive oil over medium heat.
2. Add thinly sliced onion and julienned carrots to the skillet. Sauté until the vegetables are softened.
3. Add minced garlic to the skillet and sauté for an additional 1-2 minutes until fragrant.
4. Push the vegetables to one side of the skillet and add ground turkey to the empty side. Cook the turkey, breaking it apart with a spoon, until browned.
5. Combine the shredded cabbage with the sautéed vegetables and turkey in the skillet.
6. Sprinkle dried thyme, paprika, caraway seeds, salt, and pepper over the mixture. Stir adequately to combine.
7. Cover the skillet and let the mixture cook for 15-20 minutes, stirring occasionally, until the cabbage is tender.
8. Adjust seasoning if necessary.
9. Garnish with fresh parsley if desired.
10. Serve the cabbage and turkey sauté hot.

Nutritional Information (Per Serving):

- **Carbs:** 15g
- **Sodium:** 350mg
- **Phosphorus:** 250mg
- **Potassium:** 550mg
- **Protein:** 25g

<u>Sweet Potato and Black Bean Quesadillas</u>

Prep Time: 20 minutes | Cook Time: 20 minutes | Servings: 4

Ingredients:

- 2 medium-sized sweet potatoes, peeled and diced
- 1 can (15 oz) black beans, drained and rinsed
- 1 cup corn kernels (fresh or frozen)
- 1 red onion, finely chopped
- 1 red bell pepper, diced
- 1 teaspoon ground cumin
- 1 teaspoon chili powder
- 1/2 teaspoon smoked paprika
- Salt and pepper to taste
- 8 whole wheat tortillas
- 1 cup low-fat shredded cheddar cheese
- Olive oil for cooking
- Fresh cilantro for garnish (optional)
- Greek yogurt or low-fat sour cream for serving (optional)

Instructions:

1. Place diced sweet potatoes in a pot of boiling water and cook until tender. Drain and set aside.

2. In a large mixing bowl, combine black beans, corn kernels, finely chopped red onion, diced red bell pepper, ground cumin, chili powder, smoked paprika, salt, and pepper. Mix adequately.

3. Heat olive oil in a skillet over medium heat. Add the cooked sweet potatoes to the skillet and mash them slightly with a fork.

4. Add the black bean and vegetable mixture to the skillet. Cook for 5-7 minutes, stirring occasionally, until the vegetables are tender and well combined.

5. Lay out the whole wheat tortillas on a clean surface.

6. Spoon the sweet potato and black bean mixture onto one half of each tortilla.

7. Sprinkle low-fat shredded cheddar cheese over the vegetable mixture.

8. Fold the other half of the tortilla over the filling, creating a quesadilla.

9. In the same skillet, cook the quesadillas for 2-3 minutes on each side or until the tortillas are golden brown and the cheese is melted.

10. Remove from the skillet and cut each quesadilla into wedges.

11. Garnish with fresh cilantro if desired and serve with a dollop of Greek yogurt or low-fat sour cream.

Nutritional Information (Per Serving):

- **Carbs:** 50g
- **Sodium:** 450mg
- **Phosphorus:** 350mg
- **Potassium:** 600mg
- **Protein:** 15g

Mediterranean Stuffed Portobello Mushrooms
Prep Time: 15 minutes | Cook Time: 20 minutes | Servings: 4

Ingredients:

- 4 large Portobello mushrooms, stems removed
- 1 cup quinoa, cooked
- 1 can (14 oz) chickpeas, drained and rinsed
- 1 cup cherry tomatoes, halved
- 1/2 cup Kalamata olives, sliced
- 1/2 cup red onion, finely chopped
- 2 cloves garlic, minced
- 1 teaspoon dried oregano
- 1 teaspoon dried basil
- 1/2 teaspoon dried thyme
- Salt and pepper to taste
- 4 tablespoons feta cheese, crumbled
- 2 tablespoons extra-virgin olive oil
- Fresh parsley for garnish (optional)
- Lemon wedges for serving (optional)

Instructions:

1. Preheat the oven to 375°F (190°C). Line a baking sheet with parchment paper.
2. Place the Portobello mushrooms on the prepared baking sheet, gill side up.
3. In a large bowl, combine cooked quinoa, drained chickpeas, halved cherry tomatoes, sliced Kalamata olives, finely chopped red onion, minced garlic, dried oregano, dried basil, dried thyme, salt, and pepper. Mix adequately.
4. Spoon the quinoa mixture into each Portobello mushroom, pressing it down gently.
5. Drizzle extra-virgin olive oil over the stuffed mushrooms.
6. Crumble feta cheese evenly over each stuffed mushroom.
7. Bake in the preheated oven for 20 minutes or until the mushrooms are tender.
8. Garnish with fresh parsley if desired.
9. Serve with lemon wedges on the side if desired.

Nutritional Information (Per Serving):

- **Carbs:** 45g
- **Sodium:** 450mg
- **Phosphorus:** 300mg
- **Potassium:** 800mg
- **Protein:** 15g

Chicken and Broccoli Quinoa Bowl

Prep Time: 15 minutes | Cook Time: 20 minutes | Servings: 4

Ingredients:

- 1 cup quinoa, rinsed
- 1 lb boneless, skinless chicken breasts, thinly sliced
- 4 cups broccoli florets
- 1 red bell pepper, thinly sliced
- 1/2 cup low-sodium soy sauce
- 2 tablespoons honey
- 2 tablespoons rice vinegar
- 1 tablespoon sesame oil
- 2 cloves garlic, minced
- 1 teaspoon fresh ginger, grated
- 1 tablespoon cornstarch
- 2 tablespoons water
- Sesame seeds for garnish (optional)
- Green onions, sliced, for garnish (optional)

Instructions:

1. In a medium saucepan, cook the quinoa according to package instructions. Set aside.
2. In a large skillet or wok, heat sesame oil over medium-high heat.
3. Add thinly sliced chicken breasts to the skillet and cook until browned and cooked through.
4. Add broccoli florets and thinly sliced red bell pepper to the skillet. Stir-fry for 3-4 minutes until the vegetables are tender-crisp.
5. In a bowl, whisk together low-sodium soy sauce, honey, rice vinegar, minced garlic, and grated fresh ginger.
6. Pour the soy sauce mixture over the chicken and vegetables in the skillet. Stir to coat evenly.
7. In a small bowl, mix cornstarch with water to create a slurry. Add the slurry to the skillet, stirring constantly until the sauce thickens.
8. Divide the cooked quinoa among four bowls.
9. Top the quinoa with the chicken and vegetable stir-fry.
10. Garnish with sesame seeds and sliced green onions if desired.

Nutritional Information (Per Serving):

- **Carbs:** 40g
- **Sodium:** 600mg
- **Phosphorus:** 300mg
- **Potassium:** 700mg
- **Protein:** 30g

Moroccan Lentil and Vegetable Tagine

Prep Time: 20 minutes | Cook Time: 40 minutes | Servings: 6

Ingredients:

- 1 cup dry green lentils, rinsed
- 1 large onion, finely chopped
- 3 cloves garlic, minced
- 1 sweet potato, peeled and diced
- 2 carrots, sliced
- 1 zucchini, diced
- 1 red bell pepper, diced
- 1 can (14 oz) diced tomatoes
- 3 cups vegetable broth
- 2 teaspoons ground cumin
- 1 teaspoon ground coriander
- 1 teaspoon ground cinnamon
- 1 teaspoon smoked paprika
- 1/2 teaspoon ground turmeric
- Salt and pepper to taste
- 2 tablespoons olive oil
- Fresh cilantro for garnish (optional)
- Lemon wedges for serving (optional)

Instructions:

1. In a large pot, heat olive oil over medium heat.

2. Add finely chopped onion and minced garlic to the pot. Sauté until the onion is translucent.

3. Stir in ground cumin, ground coriander, ground cinnamon, smoked paprika, ground turmeric, salt, and pepper. Cook for an additional 2 minutes until fragrant.

4. Add dry green lentils, diced sweet potato, sliced carrots, diced zucchini, and diced red bell pepper to the pot. Mix adequately.

5. Pour in diced tomatoes and vegetable broth. Bring the mixture to a boil, then reduce the heat and let it simmer for 30-35 minutes or until the lentils and vegetables are tender.

6. Adjust seasoning to taste.

7. Serve the Moroccan lentil and vegetable tagine hot, garnished with fresh cilantro and accompanied by lemon wedges if desired.

Nutritional Information (Per Serving):

- **Carbs:** 40g
- **Sodium:** 500mg
- **Phosphorus:** 250mg
- **Potassium:** 800mg
- **Protein:** 15g

Chapter 7: Snacks

Hummus and Veggie Stuffed Cucumber

Prep Time: 15 minutes | **Cook Time:** 0 minutes | **Servings:** 4

Ingredients:

- 2 large cucumbers
- 1 cup cherry tomatoes, halved
- 1/2 cup red bell pepper, diced
- 1/2 cup yellow bell pepper, diced
- 1/4 cup red onion, finely chopped
- 1/4 cup Kalamata olives, sliced
- 1 cup hummus (low-sodium if available)
- 1/4 cup feta cheese, crumbled
- 2 tablespoons fresh parsley, chopped
- Salt and pepper to taste

Instructions:

1. Wash and peel the cucumbers. Cut each cucumber in half lengthwise. Scoop out the seeds with a spoon to create a hollow center.
2. In a bowl, combine cherry tomatoes, red and yellow bell peppers, red onion, and Kalamata olives.
3. Mix the veggie filling with hummus in the bowl. Add salt and pepper to taste. Stir until well combined.
4. Spoon the hummus and veggie mixture into the hollowed-out center of each cucumber half.
5. Sprinkle crumbled feta cheese on top of each stuffed cucumber.
6. Finish by garnishing the stuffed cucumbers with fresh parsley.
7. Chill for at least 30 minutes before serving. Slice each stuffed cucumber into bite-sized pieces.

Nutritional Information (per serving):

- **Carbs:** 15g
- **Sodium:** 300mg
- **Phosphorus:** 100mg
- **Potassium:** 350mg
- **Protein:** 5g

Greek Yogurt and Berry Popsicles

Prep Time: 10 minutes | **Cook Time:** 0 minutes | **Servings:** 6

Ingredients:

- 2 cups Greek yogurt (low-fat or fat-free)

- 1 cup mixed berries (strawberries, blueberries, raspberries)

- 2 tablespoons honey

- 1 teaspoon vanilla extract

- 1/4 cup almond slices (optional, for topping)

Instructions:

1. Wash and dice the strawberries. If using larger berries like strawberries, ensure they are sliced into smaller, bite-sized pieces.

2. In a bowl, combine Greek yogurt, diced strawberries, blueberries, raspberries, honey, and vanilla extract. Stir until well incorporated.

3. For a smoother texture, you can blend the yogurt and berry mixture until smooth.

4. Spoon the yogurt and berry mixture into popsicle molds. If you don't have molds, small paper cups with popsicle sticks can be used as an alternative.

5. Sprinkle almond slices on top of each filled mold for added crunch.

6. Place the popsicle molds in the freezer and let them freeze for at least 4-6 hours or until solid.

7. Once fully frozen, run the molds under warm water for a few seconds to loosen the popsicles. Remove from the molds and serve.

Nutritional Information (per serving):

- **Carbs:** 20g

- **Sodium:** 40mg

- **Phosphorus:** 120mg

- **Potassium:** 200mg

- **Protein:** 8g

Roasted Chickpeas with Herbs

Prep Time: 10 minutes | **Cook Time:** 30 minutes | **Servings:** 4

Ingredients:

- 2 cans (15 oz each) chickpeas, drained and rinsed
- 2 tablespoons olive oil
- 1 teaspoon garlic powder
- 1 teaspoon onion powder
- 1 teaspoon dried thyme
- 1 teaspoon dried rosemary
- 1/2 teaspoon paprika
- Salt and black pepper to taste

Instructions:

1. Preheat your oven to 400°F (200°C).
2. Rinse and drain the canned chickpeas. Pat them dry using a kitchen towel.
3. In a bowl, toss chickpeas with olive oil, garlic powder, onion powder, dried thyme, dried rosemary, paprika, salt, and black pepper. Ensure the chickpeas are well-coated.
4. Spread the seasoned chickpeas in a single layer on a baking sheet.
5. Roast in the preheated oven for about 30 minutes or until the chickpeas are golden brown and crispy. Shake the pan or stir the chickpeas halfway through to ensure even roasting.
6. Allow the roasted chickpeas to cool slightly before serving.

Nutritional Information (per serving):

- **Carbs:** 30g
- **Sodium:** 480mg
- **Phosphorus:** 180mg
- **Potassium:** 330mg
- **Protein:** 12g

Edamame and Sea Salt Snack

Prep Time: 5 minutes | **Cook Time:** 5 minutes | **Servings:** 4

Ingredients:

- 2 cups frozen edamame, in pods
- 1 tablespoon olive oil
- Sea salt to taste

Instructions:

1. Bring a pot of water to a boil. Add frozen edamame pods and cook for 4-5 minutes or until tender.
2. Drain the boiled edamame in a colander and run cold water over them to stop the cooking process.
3. Once cooled, take out the edamame from the pods. Squeeze the pods, and the edamame beans should easily pop out. Discard the pods.
4. In a bowl, toss the edamame beans with olive oil until well-coated.
5. Sprinkle sea salt over the edamame and toss again to evenly distribute the salt.
6. Transfer the seasoned edamame to a serving dish and serve at room temperature.

Nutritional Information (per serving):

- **Carbs:** 9g
- **Sodium:** 5mg
- **Phosphorus:** 110mg
- **Potassium:** 150mg
- **Protein:** 8g

Whole Grain Pita with Tzatziki

Prep Time: 15 minutes | **Cook Time:** 0 minutes | **Servings:** 2

Ingredients:

- 2 whole grain pitas
- 1 cup Greek yogurt (low-fat or fat-free)
- 1 cucumber, peeled, diced
- 2 cloves garlic, minced
- 1 tablespoon fresh dill, chopped
- 1 tablespoon olive oil
- 1 teaspoon lemon juice
- Salt and black pepper to taste
- 1 medium tomato, diced
- 1/4 cup red onion, finely chopped
- 1/4 cup Kalamata olives, sliced
- 2 tablespoons feta cheese, crumbled

Instructions:

1. In a bowl, combine Greek yogurt, peeled and diced cucumber, minced garlic, chopped fresh dill, olive oil, lemon juice, salt, and black pepper. Mix adequately to create the tzatziki sauce.
2. Cut the whole grain pitas into halves and toast them lightly in a toaster or oven.
3. Spread a generous amount of tzatziki sauce inside each pita half.
4. Top the tzatziki with diced tomatoes, finely chopped red onion, Kalamata olives, and crumbled feta cheese.
5. Serve the whole grain pita with tzatziki immediately.

Nutritional Information (per serving):

- **Carbs:** 45g
- **Sodium:** 580mg
- **Phosphorus:** 280mg
- **Potassium:** 430mg
- **Protein:** 15g

Almond and Date Energy Balls

Prep Time: 15 minutes | **Cook Time:** 0 minutes | **Servings:** 12

Ingredients:

- 1 cup almonds, raw
- 1 cup pitted dates
- 1/4 cup unsweetened shredded coconut
- 1/4 cup almond butter
- 1 teaspoon vanilla extract
- 1/2 teaspoon cinnamon
- Pinch of salt

Instructions:

1. In a food processor, pulse the raw almonds until finely chopped.
2. Add the pitted dates to the food processor with the chopped almonds. Pulse until the mixture becomes sticky and holds together.
3. Add the unsweetened shredded coconut, almond butter, vanilla extract, cinnamon, and a pinch of salt to the almond and date mixture in the food processor. Pulse until well combined.
4. Take small portions of the mixture and roll them into bite-sized balls using your hands.
5. Place the almond and date energy balls in the refrigerator for at least 30 minutes to firm up.
6. Once chilled, the energy balls are ready to be served. Enjoy!

Nutritional Information (per serving - 2 balls):

- **Carbs:** 18g
- **Sodium:** 10mg
- **Phosphorus:** 85mg
- **Potassium:** 220mg
- **Protein:** 5g

Guacamole and Whole Grain Tortilla Chips

Prep Time: 15 minutes | **Cook Time:** 10 minutes | **Servings:** 4

Ingredients:

For Guacamole:

- 3 ripe avocados
- 1 medium tomato, diced
- 1/4 cup red onion, finely chopped
- 1 clove garlic, minced
- 1 lime, juiced
- 2 tablespoons fresh cilantro, chopped
- Salt and black pepper to taste

For Whole Grain Tortilla Chips:

- 4 whole grain tortillas
- Olive oil spray
- Sea salt to taste

Instructions:

Guacamole:

1. Cut the ripe avocados in half, take out the pit, and scoop the flesh into a bowl.
2. Mash the avocados with a fork until smooth or to your desired level of chunkiness.
3. To the mashed avocados, add diced tomatoes, finely chopped red onion, minced garlic, lime juice, and chopped cilantro. Season with salt and black pepper. Mix adequately.
4. Taste the guacamole and adjust salt, pepper, or lime juice as needed. Cover the bowl and refrigerate while preparing the tortilla chips.

Whole Grain Tortilla Chips:

1. Preheat the oven to 375°F (190°C).
2. Cut each whole grain tortilla into wedges.
3. Arrange the tortilla wedges on a baking sheet in a single layer.
4. Lightly spray the tortilla wedges with olive oil and sprinkle with sea salt.
5. Bake in the preheated oven for 8-10 minutes or until the tortilla chips are golden and crisp.
6. Allow the tortilla chips to cool before serving with the guacamole.

Nutritional Information (per serving):

- **Carbs:** 35g
- **Sodium:** 240mg
- **Phosphorus:** 150mg
- **Potassium:** 700mg
- **Protein:** 7g

Cottage Cheese and Pineapple Cups

Prep Time: 10 minutes | **Cook Time:** 0 minutes | **Servings:** 2

Ingredients:

- 1 cup low-fat cottage cheese
- 1 cup fresh pineapple, diced
- 1/4 cup unsalted almonds, sliced
- 1 tablespoon honey
- Fresh mint leaves for garnish

Instructions:

1. In a bowl, combine low-fat cottage cheese with diced fresh pineapple. Mix adequately.
2. Take two serving cups or bowls. Divide the cottage cheese and pineapple mixture evenly between them.
3. Sprinkle sliced unsalted almonds on top of the cottage cheese and pineapple mixture in each cup.
4. Drizzle honey over the almond-topped cottage cheese and pineapple.
5. Garnish each cup with fresh mint leaves for a burst of flavor.
6. Serve immediately and enjoy the delightful combination of cottage cheese and pineapple.

Nutritional Information (per serving):

- **Carbs:** 30g
- **Sodium:** 300mg
- **Phosphorus:** 250mg
- **Potassium:** 400mg
- **Protein:** 15g

Spicy Roasted Nuts Mix

Prep Time: 10 minutes | **Cook Time:** 15 minutes | **Servings:** 8

Ingredients:

- 2 cups mixed nuts (almonds, walnuts, cashews)
- 1 tablespoon olive oil
- 1 teaspoon ground cumin
- 1 teaspoon paprika
- 1/2 teaspoon cayenne pepper
- 1/2 teaspoon garlic powder
- 1/2 teaspoon onion powder
- 1/2 teaspoon sea salt

Instructions:

1. Preheat your oven to 350°F (175°C).
2. In a bowl, combine mixed nuts with olive oil, ground cumin, paprika, cayenne pepper, garlic powder, onion powder, and sea salt. Toss until the nuts are evenly coated with the spice mixture.
3. Spread the seasoned nuts in a single layer on a baking sheet.
4. Roast in the preheated oven for 12-15 minutes or until the nuts are golden brown, stirring halfway through to ensure even roasting.
5. Allow the spicy roasted nuts to cool on the baking sheet. They will become crunchier as they cool.
6. Once cooled, transfer the nuts to a serving bowl or an airtight container for storage.

Nutritional Information (per serving):

- **Carbs:** 6g
- **Sodium:** 75mg
- **Phosphorus:** 90mg
- **Potassium:** 200mg
- **Protein:** 5g

Greek Yogurt and Cucumber Dip

Prep Time: 10 minutes | **Cook Time:** 0 minutes | **Servings:** 6

Ingredients:

- 2 cups Greek yogurt (low-fat or fat-free)
- 1 cucumber, peeled, finely diced
- 2 cloves garlic, minced
- 1 tablespoon fresh dill, chopped
- 1 tablespoon lemon juice
- 1 tablespoon extra-virgin olive oil
- Salt and black pepper to taste

Instructions:

1. Peel the cucumber and finely dice it.
2. In a bowl, combine Greek yogurt, finely diced cucumber, minced garlic, chopped fresh dill, lemon juice, and extra-virgin olive oil.
3. Add salt and black pepper to taste. Stir the mixture until all ingredients are well combined.
4. Refrigerate the Greek yogurt and cucumber dip for at least 30 minutes to allow the flavors to meld.
5. Before serving, stir the dip again and adjust the seasoning if necessary. Serve chilled.

Nutritional Information (per serving):

- **Carbs:** 7g
- **Sodium:** 50mg
- **Phosphorus:** 85mg
- **Potassium:** 180mg
- **Protein:** 10g

<u>**Apple Slices with Almond Butter**</u>

Prep Time: 5 minutes | **Cook Time:** 0 minutes | **Servings:** 2

Ingredients:

- 2 medium apples, sliced
- 4 tablespoons almond butter
- 1 tablespoon chia seeds (optional)
- 1 teaspoon honey (optional)

Instructions:

1. Wash and slice the apples into thin, manageable slices.
2. Arrange the apple slices on a serving plate and serve with almond butter on the side.
3. If desired, drizzle honey over the apple slices and almond butter. Sprinkle chia seeds on top for added nutritional value.
4. Dip the apple slices in almond butter or spread almond butter on each slice before eating.

Nutritional Information (per serving):

- **Carbs:** 30g
- **Sodium:** 0mg
- **Phosphorus:** 90mg
- **Potassium:** 300mg
- **Protein:** 6g

Quinoa and Kale Patties

Prep Time: 20 minutes | **Cook Time:** 20 minutes | **Servings:** 4

Ingredients:

- 1 cup quinoa, cooked and cooled
- 2 cups kale, finely chopped
- 1/2 cup breadcrumbs (whole wheat for a heart-healthy option)
- 1/4 cup grated Parmesan cheese
- 2 cloves garlic, minced
- 1 teaspoon dried oregano
- 1 teaspoon dried thyme
- 2 large eggs, beaten
- Salt and black pepper to taste
- Olive oil for cooking

Instructions:

1. Cook quinoa according to package instructions. Allow it to cool to room temperature.
2. Finely chop the kale leaves, removing any tough stems.
3. In a large mixing bowl, combine cooked quinoa, chopped kale, breadcrumbs, grated Parmesan cheese, minced garlic, dried oregano, dried thyme, beaten eggs, salt, and black pepper. Mix until all ingredients are well combined.
4. Divide the mixture into 8 portions and form them into patties.
5. In a skillet, heat olive oil over medium heat. Cook the quinoa and kale patties for about 4-5 minutes on each side or until they are golden brown and cooked through.
6. Once cooked, transfer the patties to a serving plate.

Nutritional Information (per serving):

- **Carbs:** 35g
- **Sodium:** 250mg
- **Phosphorus:** 220mg
- **Potassium:** 350mg
- **Protein:** 10g

Carrot and Hummus Bites

Prep Time: 15 minutes | **Cook Time:** 0 minutes | **Servings:** 4

Ingredients:

- 4 large carrots, peeled and cut into sticks
- 1 cup hummus (low-sodium for a heart-healthy option)
- Fresh parsley for garnish

Instructions:

1. Peel the carrots and cut them into sticks, approximately 3 inches in length.
2. Arrange the carrot sticks on a serving plate. Place a bowl of low-sodium hummus alongside the carrot sticks.
3. Garnish the hummus with fresh parsley for added flavor and presentation.
4. Serve the carrot sticks with hummus as a delicious and healthy snack.

Nutritional Information (per serving):

- **Carbs:** 20g
- **Sodium:** 150mg
- **Phosphorus:** 120mg
- **Potassium:** 400mg
- **Protein:** 8g

Berry and Yogurt Parfait Pops

Prep Time: 15 minutes | **Cook Time:** 0 minutes | **Servings:** 6

Ingredients:

- 1 cup Greek yogurt (low-fat or fat-free)
- 1 cup mixed berries (strawberries, blueberries, raspberries)
- 2 tablespoons honey
- 1 teaspoon vanilla extract
- 1/2 cup granola (low-sugar for a heart-healthy option)

Instructions:

1. In a bowl, mix Greek yogurt with honey and vanilla extract until well combined.
2. In popsicle molds, layer the Greek yogurt mixture and mixed berries, creating alternating layers.
3. Insert popsicle sticks into the molds, making sure they are centered in each layer.
4. Sprinkle granola on top of the final yogurt layer in each mold.
5. Place the popsicle molds in the freezer and let them freeze for at least 4-6 hours or until solid.
6. Once fully frozen, run the molds under warm water for a few seconds to loosen the parfait popsicles. Remove from the molds and serve.

Nutritional Information (per serving):

- **Carbs:** 25g
- **Sodium:** 30mg
- **Phosphorus:** 110mg
- **Potassium:** 180mg
- **Protein:** 6g

Whole Grain Crackers with Smoked Salmon

Prep Time: 10 minutes | **Cook Time:** 0 minutes | **Servings:** 4

Ingredients:

- 24 whole grain crackers
- 4 ounces smoked salmon, thinly sliced
- 1/2 cup Greek yogurt (low-fat or fat-free)
- 1 tablespoon capers, drained
- 1 tablespoon red onion, finely chopped
- Fresh dill for garnish
- Lemon wedges for serving

Instructions:

1. Thinly slice the smoked salmon, chop the red onion finely, and drain the capers.
2. Lay out the whole grain crackers on a serving platter.
3. Spread a thin layer of low-fat or fat-free Greek yogurt on each cracker.
4. Place a slice of smoked salmon on top of the Greek yogurt on each cracker.
5. Sprinkle drained capers and finely chopped red onion evenly over the smoked salmon-topped crackers.
6. Garnish the whole grain crackers with fresh dill for added flavor.
7. Serve the smoked salmon-topped crackers with lemon wedges on the side.

Nutritional Information (per serving):

- **Carbs:** 25g
- **Sodium:** 380mg
- **Phosphorus:** 150mg
- **Potassium:** 200mg
- **Protein:** 12g

Avocado and Tomato Salsa with Whole Wheat Chips

Prep Time: 15 minutes | **Cook Time:** 10 minutes | **Servings:** 4

Ingredients:

For Salsa:

- 2 ripe avocados, diced
- 1 cup cherry tomatoes, diced
- 1/4 cup red onion, finely chopped
- 1/4 cup fresh cilantro, chopped
- 1 jalapeño, seeds removed and finely chopped
- 1 lime, juiced
- Salt to taste

For Whole Wheat Chips:

- 4 whole wheat tortillas
- Olive oil spray
- Sea salt to taste

Instructions:

For Salsa:

1. Dice the ripe avocados and place them in a mixing bowl.
2. Add diced cherry tomatoes, finely chopped red onion, chopped fresh cilantro, finely chopped jalapeño (seeds removed for less heat), and lime juice to the bowl with avocados.
3. Season the salsa with salt to taste. Gently toss the ingredients until well combined.

For Whole Wheat Chips:

1. Preheat your oven to 375°F (190°C).
2. Cut each whole wheat tortilla into wedges.
3. Arrange the tortilla wedges on a baking sheet in a single layer.
4. Lightly spray the tortilla wedges with olive oil and sprinkle with sea salt.
5. Bake in the preheated oven for 8-10 minutes or until the whole wheat chips are golden and crisp.
6. Serve the avocado and tomato salsa with the whole wheat chips.

Nutritional Information (per serving):

- **Carbs:** 30g
- **Sodium:** 380mg
- **Phosphorus:** 180mg
- **Potassium:** 550mg
- **Protein:** 6g

Trail Mix with Nuts and Dried Fruit

Prep Time: 10 minutes | **Cook Time:** 0 minutes | **Servings:** 8

Ingredients:

- 1 cup almonds, raw
- 1 cup walnuts, raw
- 1 cup pistachios, raw and shelled
- 1 cup dried cranberries
- 1/2 cup raisins
- 1/2 cup dried apricots, chopped
- 1/2 cup dark chocolate chips (70% cocoa or higher)
- 1/2 teaspoon sea salt

Instructions:

1. If not already shelled, shell the pistachios. Leave the almonds and walnuts raw.
2. In a large bowl, combine raw almonds, raw walnuts, shelled pistachios, dried cranberries, raisins, chopped dried apricots, and dark chocolate chips.
3. Sprinkle sea salt over the trail mix. Toss the ingredients until well combined.
4. Divide the trail mix into individual servings or store in an airtight container for later use.

Nutritional Information (per serving):

- **Carbs:** 25g
- **Sodium:** 75mg
- **Phosphorus:** 120mg
- **Potassium:** 250mg
- **Protein:** 7g

Chapter 8: Desserts

Dark Chocolate and Berry Bark

Prep Time: 15 minutes | **Cook Time:** 10 minutes | **Servings:** 12

Ingredients:

- 8 ounces dark chocolate, chopped

- 1 cup dried mixed berries (such as blueberries, cranberries, and cherries)

- 1/4 cup unsalted almonds, chopped

- 1/4 cup unsalted pistachios, chopped

- 1/4 cup unsweetened shredded coconut

Instructions:

1. Line a baking sheet with parchment paper.

2. In a heatproof bowl, melt the dark chocolate using a double boiler or microwave in 30-second intervals, stirring until smooth.

3. Once the chocolate is melted, spread it evenly onto the prepared baking sheet.

4. Sprinkle the mixed berries, chopped almonds, chopped pistachios, and shredded coconut evenly over the melted chocolate.

5. Place the baking sheet in the refrigerator for at least 1 hour or until the chocolate is set.

6. Once the chocolate has hardened, break it into pieces of your desired size.

7. Store the dark chocolate and berry bark in an airtight container in the refrigerator.

Nutritional Information (per serving):

- **Carbs:** 15g

- **Sodium:** 5mg

- **Phosphorus:** 30mg

- **Potassium:** 100mg

- **Protein:** 2g

Greek Yogurt and Honey Frozen Bites

Prep Time: 10 minutes | **Freeze Time:** 2 hours | **Servings:** 6

Ingredients:

- 2 cups plain Greek yogurt

- 1/4 cup honey

- 1 cup mixed berries (such as strawberries, blueberries, and raspberries), diced

- 1/4 cup unsalted almonds, sliced

Instructions:

1. In a mixing bowl, put together the plain Greek yogurt and honey. Stir until well combined.

2. Fold in the diced mixed berries and sliced almonds into the yogurt mixture.

3. Spoon the mixture into silicone ice cube trays or small molds, distributing it evenly.

4. Place the trays or molds in the freezer and let the bites freeze for at least 2 hours or until solid.

5. Once frozen, pop the yogurt bites out of the molds.

6. Serve immediately or store in an airtight container in the freezer.

Nutritional Information (per serving):

- **Carbs:** 15g

- **Sodium:** 20mg

- **Phosphorus:** 100mg

- **Potassium:** 150mg

- **Protein:** 8g

Lemon Blueberry Chia Seed Pudding

Prep Time: 10 minutes | **Chill Time:** 4 hours or overnight | **Servings:** 4

Ingredients:

- 1 cup unsweetened almond milk
- 1/4 cup chia seeds
- 2 tablespoons maple syrup
- 1 teaspoon vanilla extract
- Zest of 1 lemon
- 1 cup fresh blueberries, washed and halved

Instructions:

1. In a mixing bowl, whisk together the unsweetened almond milk, chia seeds, maple syrup, vanilla extract, and lemon zest.
2. Allow the mixture to sit for a few minutes, then whisk again to prevent clumps.
3. Gently fold in the fresh blueberries into the chia seed mixture.
4. Divide the mixture evenly among four serving glasses or jars.
5. Refrigerate the pudding for at least 4 hours or overnight to allow the chia seeds to expand and create a pudding-like consistency.
6. Before serving, give the pudding a good stir and top with additional blueberries if desired.

Nutritional Information (per serving):

- **Carbs:** 20g
- **Sodium:** 20mg
- **Phosphorus:** 100mg
- **Potassium:** 150mg
- **Protein:** 4g

Almond Flour Banana Muffins

Prep Time: 15 minutes | **Cook Time:** 20 minutes | **Servings:** 12

Ingredients:

- 2 cups almond flour
- 1 teaspoon baking powder
- 1/2 teaspoon baking soda
- 1/4 teaspoon salt
- 3 ripe bananas, mashed
- 3 large eggs
- 1/4 cup coconut oil, melted
- 1 teaspoon vanilla extract
- 1/2 cup chopped walnuts (optional)

Instructions:

1. Preheat the oven to 350°F (175°C). Line a muffin tin with paper liners.
2. In a large bowl, put together the almond flour, baking powder, baking soda, and salt.
3. In a separate bowl, mix the mashed bananas, eggs, melted coconut oil, and vanilla extract.
4. Add the wet ingredients to the dry ingredients, stirring until just combined. If using, fold in the chopped walnuts.
5. Spoon the batter into the muffin cups, filling each about 2/3 full.
6. Bake for 18-20 minutes or until a toothpick inserted into the center of a muffin comes out clean.
7. Allow the muffins to cool in the tin for 5 minutes, then transfer them to a wire rack to cool completely.

Nutritional Information (per muffin):

- **Carbs:** 10g
- **Sodium:** 130mg
- **Phosphorus:** 70mg
- **Potassium:** 180mg
- **Protein:** 5g

Berry and Oat Crumble Bars

Prep Time: 15 minutes | **Bake Time:** 35 minutes | **Servings:** 12

Ingredients:

For the Berry Filling:

- 2 cups mixed berries (such as strawberries, blueberries, and raspberries)
- 1/4 cup maple syrup
- 2 tablespoons chia seeds

For the Oat Crumble:

- 1 cup old-fashioned oats
- 1/2 cup almond flour
- 1/4 cup coconut oil, melted
- 1/4 cup maple syrup
- 1/2 teaspoon vanilla extract
- 1/4 teaspoon salt

Instructions:

1. Preheat the oven to 350°F (175°C). Line a square baking pan with parchment paper, leaving some overhang on the sides for easy removal.

2. In a medium saucepan, put together the mixed berries, maple syrup, and chia seeds. Cook over medium heat, stirring occasionally, until the berries break down and the mixture thickens (about 5-7 minutes). Remove from heat and let it cool.

3. In a large mixing bowl, put together the old-fashioned oats, almond flour, melted coconut oil, maple syrup, vanilla extract, and salt. Mix until the ingredients are well combined.

4. Press two-thirds of the oat mixture into the bottom of the prepared baking pan to create the base.

5. Spread the cooled berry filling evenly over the oat base.

6. Sprinkle the remaining oat mixture over the berry filling, creating a crumble topping.

7. Bake in the preheated oven for 35 minutes or until the edges are golden brown.

8. Allow the bars to cool completely in the pan before using the parchment paper overhang to lift them out. Cut into squares.

Nutritional Information (per serving):

- **Carbs:** 25g
- **Sodium:** 20mg
- **Phosphorus:** 60mg
- **Potassium:** 120mg
- **Protein:** 3g

Chocolate Avocado Mousse

Prep Time: 10 minutes | **Chill Time:** 2 hours | **Servings:** 4

Ingredients:

- 2 ripe avocados, peeled and pitted
- 1/2 cup unsweetened cocoa powder
- 1/2 cup maple syrup
- 1/3 cup unsweetened almond milk
- 1 teaspoon vanilla extract
- A pinch of salt
- Fresh berries for garnish (optional)

Instructions:

1. In a food processor, put together the ripe avocados, unsweetened cocoa powder, maple syrup, unsweetened almond milk, vanilla extract, and a pinch of salt.
2. Blend the ingredients until smooth and creamy, scraping down the sides of the processor bowl as needed.
3. Taste the mousse and adjust sweetness if necessary by adding more maple syrup.
4. Once smooth, transfer the mousse to serving glasses or bowls.
5. Refrigerate the mousse for at least 2 hours to allow it to set.
6. Before serving, garnish with fresh berries if desired.

Nutritional Information (per serving):

- **Carbs:** 25g
- **Sodium:** 5mg
- **Phosphorus:** 120mg
- **Potassium:** 600mg
- **Protein:** 4g

Coconut and Mango Sorbet

Prep Time: 15 minutes | **Freeze Time:** 4 hours | **Servings:** 6

Ingredients:

- 2 cups ripe mango, peeled and diced
- 1 can (14 ounces) coconut milk
- 1/2 cup honey
- Juice of 1 lime
- 1/4 cup shredded coconut (optional)

Instructions:

1. In a blender, put together the diced ripe mango, coconut milk, honey, and lime juice.
2. Blend until smooth and well combined.
3. If desired, fold in the shredded coconut into the sorbet mixture.
4. Pour the mixture into a shallow dish, spreading it evenly.
5. Place the dish in the freezer and let it freeze for about 4 hours, or until the sorbet is firm.
6. Every hour during the freezing process, stir the sorbet with a fork to prevent ice crystals from forming.
7. Once the sorbet is fully frozen and has a smooth texture, it's ready to serve.
8. Scoop the sorbet into bowls or cones, and enjoy!

Nutritional Information (per serving):

- **Carbs:** 40g
- **Sodium:** 10mg
- **Phosphorus:** 80mg
- **Potassium:** 300mg
- **Protein:** 2g

Pistachio and Date Energy Bites

Prep Time: 15 minutes | **Chill Time:** 30 minutes | **Servings:** 12

Ingredients:

- 1 cup pitted dates, chopped
- 1 cup roasted unsalted pistachios
- 1/4 cup rolled oats
- 2 tablespoons chia seeds
- 1/2 teaspoon vanilla extract
- A pinch of salt
- Shredded coconut for rolling (optional)

Instructions:

1. In a food processor, put together the chopped pitted dates, roasted unsalted pistachios, rolled oats, chia seeds, vanilla extract, and a pinch of salt.
2. Pulse the ingredients until they form a sticky and uniform mixture.
3. Scoop out portions of the mixture and roll them into bite-sized balls using your hands.
4. If desired, roll each energy bite in shredded coconut for an extra layer of flavor.
5. Place the energy bites on a tray or plate and refrigerate for at least 30 minutes to firm up.
6. Once chilled, transfer the energy bites to an airtight container and store in the refrigerator.

Nutritional Information (per serving):

- **Carbs:** 20g
- **Sodium:** 10mg
- **Phosphorus:** 80mg
- **Potassium:** 250mg
- **Protein:** 4g

<u>Orange and Walnut Quinoa Cookies</u>

Prep Time: 15 minutes | **Bake Time:** 12 minutes | **Servings:** 18

Ingredients:

- 1 cup cooked quinoa, cooled
- 1 cup whole wheat flour
- 1/2 cup unsalted butter, softened
- 1/2 cup pure maple syrup
- Zest of 1 orange
- 2 tablespoons fresh orange juice
- 1 teaspoon vanilla extract
- 1/2 cup chopped walnuts
- 1/2 teaspoon baking powder
- A pinch of salt

Instructions:

1. Preheat the oven to 350°F (175°C). Line a baking sheet with parchment paper.
2. In a large bowl, cream together the softened unsalted butter and pure maple syrup until well combined.
3. Add the cooled, cooked quinoa, whole wheat flour, orange zest, fresh orange juice, and vanilla extract to the butter and syrup mixture. Mix until a dough forms.
4. Fold in the chopped walnuts, baking powder, and a pinch of salt into the cookie dough.
5. Using a cookie scoop or spoon, drop rounded balls of dough onto the prepared baking sheet, spacing them about 2 inches apart.
6. Flatten each cookie slightly with the back of a spoon.
7. Bake in the preheated oven for approximately 12 minutes or until the edges are golden brown.
8. Allow the cookies to cool on the baking sheet for a few minutes before transferring them to a wire rack to cool completely.

Nutritional Information (per serving - 1 cookie):

- **Carbs:** 15g
- **Sodium:** 20mg
- **Phosphorus:** 60mg
- **Potassium:** 80mg
- **Protein:** 2g

<u>Cinnamon Baked Apples</u>

Prep Time: 15 minutes | **Bake Time:** 30 minutes | **Servings:** 4

Ingredients:

- 4 large apples, cored and sliced
- 2 tablespoons pure maple syrup
- 1 tablespoon lemon juice
- 1 teaspoon ground cinnamon
- 1/4 teaspoon nutmeg
- 1/4 cup chopped walnuts
- 1 tablespoon unsalted butter, diced

Instructions:

1. Preheat the oven to 375°F (190°C). Grease a baking dish with a little bit of butter.
2. In a bowl, toss the cored and sliced apples with pure maple syrup, lemon juice, ground cinnamon, and nutmeg until the apples are evenly coated.
3. Transfer the coated apples to the prepared baking dish, spreading them out in an even layer.
4. Sprinkle the chopped walnuts over the apples.
5. Dot the top of the apples with diced unsalted butter.
6. Bake in the preheated oven for about 30 minutes or until the apples are tender and the edges are golden.
7. Remove from the oven and let the baked apples cool for a few minutes before serving.

Nutritional Information (per serving):

- **Carbs:** 30g
- **Sodium:** 0mg
- **Phosphorus:** 20mg
- **Potassium:** 200mg
- **Protein:** 1g

Raspberry Almond Chia Seed Parfait

Prep Time: 15 minutes | **Chill Time:** 2 hours | **Servings:** 2

Ingredients:

- 1 cup unsweetened almond milk
- 1/4 cup chia seeds
- 2 tablespoons pure maple syrup
- 1/2 teaspoon almond extract
- 1 cup fresh raspberries
- 1/4 cup sliced almonds
- Greek yogurt for layering (optional)

Instructions:

1. In a bowl, whisk together the unsweetened almond milk, chia seeds, pure maple syrup, and almond extract. Make sure the mixture is well combined.

2. Let the chia seed mixture sit for a few minutes, then whisk again to avoid clumping. Repeat this process a couple of times over 10-15 minutes.

3. Cover the bowl and refrigerate the chia seed mixture for at least 2 hours or overnight to allow it to thicken.

4. Before assembling the parfait, stir the chia seed mixture to ensure a smooth consistency.

5. In serving glasses or bowls, layer the chia seed mixture with fresh raspberries and sliced almonds. If desired, add a layer of Greek yogurt.

6. Repeat the layering until the glasses are filled.

7. Top the parfait with additional raspberries and sliced almonds.

8. Refrigerate for a little while longer if desired or serve immediately.

Nutritional Information (per serving):

- **Carbs:** 25g
- **Sodium:** 30mg
- **Phosphorus:** 120mg
- **Potassium:** 250mg
- **Protein:** 6g

Whole Wheat Chocolate Chip Cookies

Prep Time: 15 minutes | **Bake Time:** 10 minutes | **Servings:** 24

Ingredients:

- 1 cup whole wheat flour
- 1/2 cup unsalted butter, softened
- 1/2 cup pure maple syrup
- 1 large egg
- 1 teaspoon vanilla extract
- 1/2 teaspoon baking soda
- 1/4 teaspoon salt
- 1 cup dark chocolate chips
- 1/2 cup chopped walnuts (optional)

Instructions:

1. Preheat the oven to 350°F (175°C). Line a baking sheet with parchment paper.
2. In a bowl, cream together the softened unsalted butter and pure maple syrup until smooth.
3. Add the egg and vanilla extract to the butter and syrup mixture. Mix until well combined.
4. In a separate bowl, whisk together the whole wheat flour, baking soda, and salt.
5. Gradually add the dry ingredients to the wet ingredients, mixing until a cookie dough forms.
6. Fold in the dark chocolate chips and chopped walnuts (if using).
7. Drop rounded tablespoons of dough onto the prepared baking sheet, spacing them about 2 inches apart.
8. Bake in the preheated oven for approximately 10 minutes or until the edges are golden brown.
9. Allow the cookies to cool on the baking sheet for a few minutes before transferring them to a wire rack to cool completely.

Nutritional Information (per serving - 1 cookie):

- **Carbs:** 15g
- **Sodium:** 35mg
- **Phosphorus:** 50mg
- **Potassium:** 70mg
- **Protein:** 2g

Vanilla Bean and Berry Popsicles

Prep Time: 10 minutes | **Freeze Time:** 4 hours | **Servings:** 6

Ingredients:

- 2 cups mixed berries (such as strawberries, blueberries, and raspberries)
- 1 vanilla bean
- 1/4 cup honey
- 2 cups plain Greek yogurt
- 1/4 cup sliced almonds

Instructions:

1. Wash and prepare the mixed berries. If using strawberries, hull and slice them.
2. Split the vanilla bean lengthwise and scrape out the seeds.
3. In a bowl, put together the mixed berries, vanilla bean seeds, and honey. Toss until the berries are coated in the vanilla-infused honey.
4. In a separate bowl, mix the plain Greek yogurt until smooth.
5. Layer the mixed berries and vanilla honey mixture with the Greek yogurt in popsicle molds.
6. Insert popsicle sticks and freeze for at least 4 hours or until fully set.
7. Before serving, sprinkle sliced almonds onto each popsicle.
8. To remove the popsicles from the molds, briefly run them under warm water.

Nutritional Information (per serving):

- **Carbs:** 20g
- **Sodium:** 30mg
- **Phosphorus:** 100mg
- **Potassium:** 200mg
- **Protein:** 5g

Pumpkin and Pecan Baked Oatmeal

Prep Time: 15 minutes | **Bake Time:** 40 minutes | **Servings:** 8

Ingredients:

- 2 cups old-fashioned oats
- 1/2 cup chopped pecans
- 1 teaspoon baking powder
- 1/2 teaspoon ground cinnamon
- 1/4 teaspoon nutmeg
- 1/4 teaspoon salt
- 1 1/2 cups unsweetened almond milk
- 1/2 cup pure pumpkin puree
- 1/4 cup pure maple syrup
- 2 large eggs
- 1 teaspoon vanilla extract

Instructions:

1. Preheat the oven to 350°F (175°C). Grease a baking dish with a little bit of oil.
2. In a bowl, put together the old-fashioned oats, chopped pecans, baking powder, ground cinnamon, nutmeg, and salt.
3. In a separate bowl, whisk together the unsweetened almond milk, pure pumpkin puree, pure maple syrup, eggs, and vanilla extract.
4. Pour the wet ingredients into the dry ingredients and stir until well combined.
5. Transfer the mixture to the prepared baking dish, spreading it out evenly.
6. Bake in the preheated oven for approximately 40 minutes or until the edges are golden brown and the center is set.
7. Allow the baked oatmeal to cool for a few minutes before slicing.

Nutritional Information (per serving):

- **Carbs:** 30g
- **Sodium:** 120mg
- **Phosphorus:** 100mg
- **Potassium:** 180mg
- **Protein:** 6g

Greek Yogurt and Berry Tart

Prep Time: 20 minutes | **Chill Time:** 2 hours | **Servings:** 8

Ingredients:

For the Crust:

- 1 1/2 cups almond flour
- 1/4 cup coconut oil, melted
- 2 tablespoons pure maple syrup
- 1/2 teaspoon vanilla extract
- A pinch of salt

For the Filling:

- 2 cups Greek yogurt
- 1/4 cup honey
- 1 teaspoon vanilla extract

For the Topping:

- 1 cup mixed berries (such as blueberries, raspberries, and strawberries)
- 1 tablespoon fresh mint leaves, thinly sliced

Instructions:

Crust:

1. Preheat the oven to 350°F (175°C). Grease a tart pan with a removable bottom.

2. In a bowl, put together the almond flour, melted coconut oil, pure maple syrup, vanilla extract, and a pinch of salt.

3. Press the mixture into the bottom of the tart pan, creating an even crust.

4. Bake the crust in the preheated oven for about 10 minutes or until lightly golden. Allow it to cool completely.

Filling:

5. In a separate bowl, mix together the Greek yogurt, honey, and vanilla extract.

6. Spread the Greek yogurt mixture evenly over the cooled almond crust.

Topping:

7. Arrange the mixed berries on top of the Greek yogurt filling.

8. Sprinkle the thinly sliced fresh mint leaves over the berries.

9. Refrigerate the tart for at least 2 hours before serving to allow it to set.

Nutritional Information (per serving):

- **Carbs:** 25g
- **Sodium:** 20mg
- **Phosphorus:** 150mg
- **Potassium:** 200mg
- **Protein:** 8g

Quinoa and Coconut Pudding

Prep Time: 10 minutes | **Cook Time:** 25 minutes | **Servings:** 4

Ingredients:

- 1/2 cup quinoa, rinsed
- 1 can (14 ounces) light coconut milk
- 1/4 cup honey
- 1/2 teaspoon vanilla extract
- 1/4 cup shredded coconut
- Fresh berries for garnish (optional)
- Mint leaves for garnish (optional)

Instructions:

1. In a medium-sized saucepan, put together the rinsed quinoa, light coconut milk, honey, and vanilla extract.
2. Bring the mixture to a boil over medium heat. Once boiling, reduce the heat to low, cover, and simmer for 20-25 minutes or until the quinoa is cooked and has absorbed most of the coconut milk.
3. Stir in the shredded coconut during the last 5 minutes of cooking.
4. Take out the saucepan from heat and let the quinoa pudding sit, covered, for an additional 5 minutes to absorb any remaining liquid.
5. Fluff the quinoa pudding with a fork and spoon it into serving bowls.
6. Garnish with fresh berries and mint leaves if desired.
7. Serve warm or chilled.

Nutritional Information (per serving):

- **Carbs:** 40g
- **Sodium:** 20mg
- **Phosphorus:** 150mg
- **Potassium:** 200mg
- **Protein:** 5g

<u>Walnut and Fig Energy Bars</u>

Prep Time: 15 minutes | **Chill Time:** 1 hour | **Servings:** 12

Ingredients:

- 1 cup dried figs, stemmed and chopped
- 1 cup walnuts
- 1/2 cup rolled oats
- 1/4 cup chia seeds
- 1/4 cup honey
- 1/2 teaspoon vanilla extract
- A pinch of salt

Instructions:

1. In a food processor, put together the dried figs, walnuts, rolled oats, chia seeds, honey, vanilla extract, and a pinch of salt.
2. Process the mixture until it forms a sticky dough that holds together when pressed.
3. Line a square baking dish with parchment paper, leaving some overhang on the sides for easy removal.
4. Transfer the fig and walnut mixture to the baking dish, spreading it out evenly.
5. Press the mixture down firmly to create a compact and even layer.
6. Refrigerate the mixture for at least 1 hour to firm up.
7. Once chilled, use the parchment paper overhang to lift the mixture out of the dish.
8. Cut into bars of your desired size.
9. Store the energy bars in an airtight container in the refrigerator.

Nutritional Information (per serving):

- **Carbs:** 20g
- **Sodium:** 5mg
- **Phosphorus:** 80mg
- **Potassium:** 200mg
- **Protein:** 3g

Frozen Banana and Almond Butter Bites

Prep Time: 10 minutes | **Freeze Time:** 2 hours | **Servings:** 4

Ingredients:

- 2 large bananas, peeled and sliced
- 1/4 cup almond butter
- 1/4 cup dark chocolate chips
- 1/4 cup chopped almonds
- 1 tablespoon coconut oil
- A pinch of sea salt

Instructions:

1. Line a tray or plate that fits in your freezer with parchment paper.
2. Slice the bananas into rounds and arrange half of them on the prepared tray.
3. In a small saucepan over low heat, melt the almond butter, dark chocolate chips, coconut oil, and a pinch of sea salt. Stir until smooth and well combined.
4. Spoon a small amount of the almond butter and chocolate mixture onto each banana slice.
5. Place another banana slice on top, creating a "sandwich."
6. Repeat the process with the remaining banana slices.
7. Sprinkle chopped almonds over the top of each banana "sandwich."
8. Place the tray in the freezer and freeze for at least 2 hours or until the bites are completely frozen.
9. Once frozen, transfer the banana and almond butter bites to an airtight container and store in the freezer.

Nutritional Information (per serving):

- **Carbs:** 30g
- **Sodium:** 5mg
- **Phosphorus:** 100mg
- **Potassium:** 400mg
- **Protein:** 4g

Chapter 9: Tips for Healthy Aging

Staying Active

Regular exercise is a must for staying healthy and vibrant as we age. It's not just about keeping the heart in good shape; it also boosts energy, improves mobility, and supports mental well-being. Adding physical activity to daily routines can significantly impact seniors' health and quality of life.

Activities Perfect for Seniors

- **Walking:** It's a low-impact exercise that you can do almost anywhere. Try to walk briskly for at least 30 minutes most days of the week.

- **Swimming:** Gentle on the joints, swimming and water aerobics are fantastic for cardiovascular health and muscle strength.

- **Yoga and Tai Chi:** These practices help with flexibility, balance, and mental focus, which reduces the risk of falls and promotes relaxation.

- **Strength Training:** Light weightlifting or using resistance bands can help maintain muscle mass and bone density. Aim to work on major muscle groups twice a week.

Staying Hydrated

Keeping hydrated is crucial for overall health, especially for seniors, who are more prone to dehydration. Proper hydration aids digestion, circulation, temperature regulation, and cognitive function.

Tips for Staying Hydrated:

- **Drink Water Regularly:** Aim for at least 8 cups of water daily. Keep a water bottle with you and take small sips throughout the day.

- **Eat Hydrating Foods:** Incorporate fruits and veggies with high water content, like cucumbers, melons, oranges, and strawberries.

- **Monitor Fluid Intake:** Listen to your body. Thirst, dry mouth, dark urine, and fatigue can all be signs of dehydration.

- **Limit Dehydrating Beverages:** Cut down on caffeinated and alcoholic drinks, as they can lead to dehydration.

Managing Dietary Restrictions

Many seniors have specific dietary needs due to conditions like diabetes, heart disease, or kidney issues. Balancing these restrictions while still enjoying a varied diet is crucial in maintaining health and enjoying your meals.

Strategies for Managing Dietary Restrictions:

- **Mindful Eating:** Focus on the eating experience. Savor each bite, eat slowly, and pay attention to hunger and fullness cues. This can help prevent overeating and increase satisfaction.

- **Portion Control:** Use smaller plates and bowls to help manage portion sizes. Pay attention to serving sizes on food labels and be mindful of portions at restaurants.

- **Customized Meal Planning:** Adapt recipes to meet dietary needs by substituting ingredients or adjusting seasonings. For example, use herbs and spices instead of salt for flavor, or choose whole grains over refined grains.

- **Regular Monitoring:** Keep track of what you eat and monitor any health changes. Consult with a healthcare provider or dietitian for personalized advice and adjustments.

Embracing Mindful Eating

Mindful eating is all about being aware and appreciating your food. It means paying full attention to the eating experience, from preparation to the actual meal, and recognizing your body's hunger and satiety signals.

Techniques for Mindful Eating:

- **Eliminate Distractions:** Turn off the TV, put away devices, and focus on your meal. Eating without distractions helps you enjoy your food and notice when you're full.

- **Chew Thoroughly:** Take your time to chew each bite well. This not only helps with digestion but also lets you fully appreciate the flavors and textures.

- **Appreciate Your Food:** Before eating, take a moment to appreciate your food. Consider its origins, the effort that went into preparing it, and the nutritional benefits it offers.

- **Listen to Your Body:** Pay attention to your hunger and fullness cues. Eat when you're hungry and stop when you're comfortably full, even if there's food left on your plate.

By integrating these healthy aging tips into your daily routine, you can enhance your physical and mental well-being and make the most of your senior years with vitality and joy.

Conclusion

Thank you for exploring "The Ultimate DASH Diet Cookbook for Seniors." We trust that this cookbook has equipped you with the knowledge, motivation, and practical tools to fully embrace the DASH diet and improve your overall well-being.

Reflecting on Your Journey

Through your exploration of the different chapters, you have gained valuable insights into the significance of the DASH diet, its benefits for older adults, and practical ways to integrate it into your everyday routine. From understanding the essential nutrients that support healthy aging to discovering delicious and easy-to-prepare recipes, you've taken significant steps toward a healthier lifestyle.

Celebrating Your Progress

Embracing a different approach to eating is a transformative experience, and each minor adjustment you make is an achievement worthy of recognition. Whether you've discovered the pleasure of experimenting with new recipes, realized the benefits of staying hydrated, or embraced physical activities that promote an active lifestyle, these efforts contribute to a healthier, happier you. It's important to recognize and value your progress as you go.

Anticipating the Future

The DASH diet offers a sustainable and fun approach to eating that can support your health for years to come. As you continue exploring and experimenting with the recipes and tips in this cookbook, you'll discover that maintaining a nutritious diet becomes effortless.

Your Health, Your Future

Your commitment to adopting the DASH diet demonstrates your dedication to maintaining a vibrant and healthy lifestyle. By prioritizing the DASH diet, you are making a valuable investment in your future and ensuring that you stay healthy to enjoy the many beautiful moments ahead.

Thank you for choosing *"The Complete DASH Diet Cookbook for Seniors"* as your trusted companion. We hope it continues to be a valuable resource and a wellspring of inspiration. Here's to a future filled with delectable meals, robust health, and the happiness that stems from self-care.

Here's to wishing you all the best as you embark on your journey towards a healthier and happier life!

Recipes Index